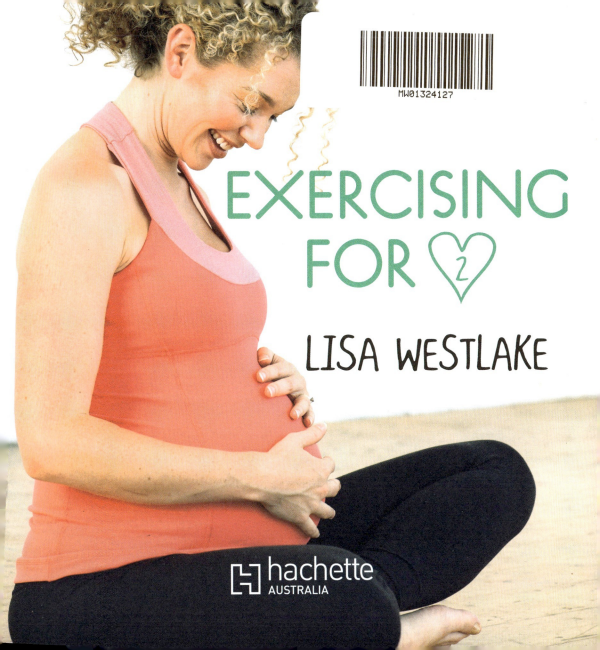

AN IMPORTANT NOTE
The exercises in this book are designed as low-intensity, low-impact programs suitable for most pregnant women with a low-risk, healthy pregnancy. If you have a history of preterm labour or certain medical conditions, including poorly controlled diabetes, high blood pressure, heart disease and placenta praevia, you will need to be especially careful. Before undertaking any prenatal exercises, programs or classes always consult your doctor or midwife for a prenatal screening and only commence exercising that is compatible with your particular health situation and needs with their consent. Although every effort has been made to ensure that the contents of this book are accurate, it must not be treated as a substitute for qualified medical advice. To minimise the risk of incident/injury carefully read the information in parts one and two of this book, which contain critical information on important health considerations and safe exercising guidelines. Neither the author nor the publisher can be held responsible for any loss or claim arising out of the use, or misuse, of the suggestions made or the failure to take medical advice.

hachette
AUSTRALIA

Published in Australia and New Zealand in 2011
by Hachette Australia
(an imprint of Hachette Australia Pty Limited)
Level 17, 207 Kent Street, Sydney NSW 2000
www.hachette.com.au

10 9 8 7 6 5 4 3 2 1

Copyright © Lisa Westlake 2011

This book is copyright. Apart from any fair dealing for the purposes of private study, research, criticism or review permitted under the Copyright Act 1968, no part may be stored or reproduced by any process without prior written permission. Enquiries should be made to the publisher.

Cataloguing-in-Publication data for this book is available from the National Library of Australia

ISBN 978 0 7336 2503 9

Photography by Bronwyn Kidd
Cover design by Christabella Designs
Text design by Agave Creative
Typeset in Avenir by Agave Creative Group
Printed in China by South China Printing Co. Ltd.

Hachette Australia's policy is to use papers that are natural, renewable and recyclable products and made from wood grown in sustainable forests. The logging and manufacturing processes are expected to conform to the environmental regulations of the country of origin.

Author's Note

Pregnancy is an exciting time. It is a time when women take the opportunity to focus on lifestyle, exercise and well-being, to nurture themselves and their baby.

Exercising for Two will help you understand all that is going on in your body and show you how you can reap the benefits of safe and appropriate exercise during this very special time. Every woman and every pregnancy is different, so *Exercising for Two* outlines all the considerations of individual exercise selection and allows you to custom design your program to suit your fitness, pregnancy, and specific needs.

There is an element of controversy in several areas relating to prenatal fitness guidelines. Expert opinions vary about issues such as safe exercise positioning and intensity. Research outcomes lack consensus and there is certainly room for further study. I believe that it is wiser to err on the side of caution. My philosophy is 'if in doubt, leave it out', so I make no apology for taking the conservative and more commonly considered correct approach in *Exercising for Two's* exercise prescription and advice. The recommendations are also in keeping with the revised American College of Obstetric and Gynaecology exercise during pregnancy guidelines.

Safe and appropriate exercise is the all-important focus. Choosing sensible exercise is vital to a healthy and comfortable pregnancy, delivery and outcome. The right exercise will not be detrimental to the health of mum or bub, nor cause unwanted aches, pains or regrets.

Know your body, listen to your body and enjoy the results

contents

Congratulations 6

PART ONE – GETTING STARTED

How to use this book 10
You are unique 11
The benefits of prenatal exercise 12
Before you start 14
Can exercise harm me and my baby? 16
Why you need to modify your exercise 19
When you need to take extra care and modify your exercise further 30
Choose exercises that suit you and your baby 37
Nutrition 44
Your 9-month workout 45

PART TWO – EXERCISING FOR TWO BASICS

Pregnancy fitness fundamentals 54
Listening to your body 63

PART THREE – THE EXERCISES

Safe and effective exercise 68
Mobility exercises 70
Pelvic floor training 89
Posture 98
Core strength and stability 100
Cardiovascular training 117
Strength exercises 135
Aqua exercise 176
Labour preparation 180
Stretch and mobilise 188
Relaxation 195
Getting ready for B-day 199
Early days of motherhood 203

PART FOUR – THE EXERCISE PROGRAMS

Exercise programs 206
Thank you 215

congratulations

A precious time of growth, development and preparation

Pregnancy is an amazing time in a woman's life. It is also a time where women take this opportunity to focus on lifestyle, exercise and well-being to nurture themselves and their baby-to-be.

This is the book I've dreamt of writing for many years; on a topic I am incredibly passionate about – helping women enjoy safe and appropriate exercise so that they feel their physical and emotional best during pregnancy.

Exercising for Two is a culmination of more than two decades of working with pregnant women, mums and their babies, and many wonderful women's health professionals. Combining my experiences as a physiotherapist and fitness instructor has allowed me to work with people of all ages, stages and fitness levels to provide custom designed prenatal and postnatal exercise programs that allow women to safely and confidently improve their health and well-being. As a result of my working with women in my physiotherapy fitness classes, I have had the pleasure of hearing what mums-to-be need, want and hope for. Together we have shared tears, laughter and joy. My own pregnancies, deliveries and experiences of early motherhood have only added to my desire to write this book.

There are so many myths out there about what to do and what not to do during your pregnancy. My aim is to give sound advice to help guide you through an exercise program that is not only adjusted to each stage of your pregnancy but will also help you to get ready, emotionally and physically, for labour.

As a fitness professional I hope you discover and enjoy the benefits of exercises that suit your pregnancy and your lifestyle.

As a physiotherapist I encourage you to focus on the big picture of long-term health and well-being for you and your baby. Welcome and acknowledge the changes of pregnancy and be prepared to adapt your fitness training accordingly. Above all, listen to your body.

As a mother I hope you can relish the joy of the journey and the magic of the miracle.

Enjoy this wonderful time in your life.

Lisa Westlake

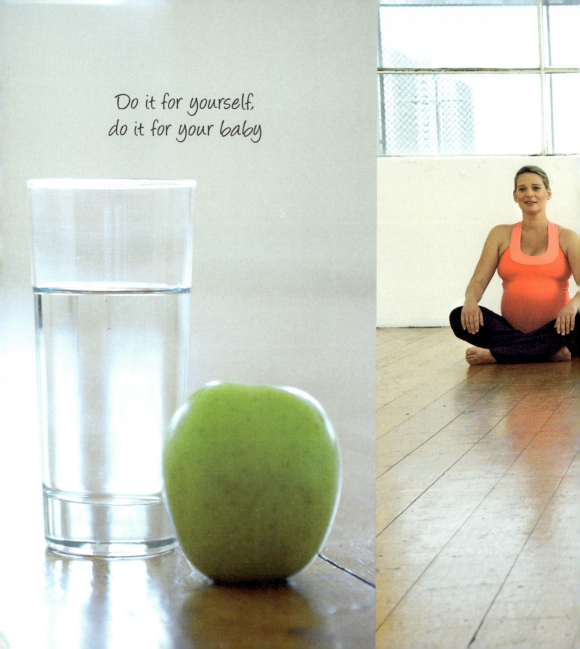

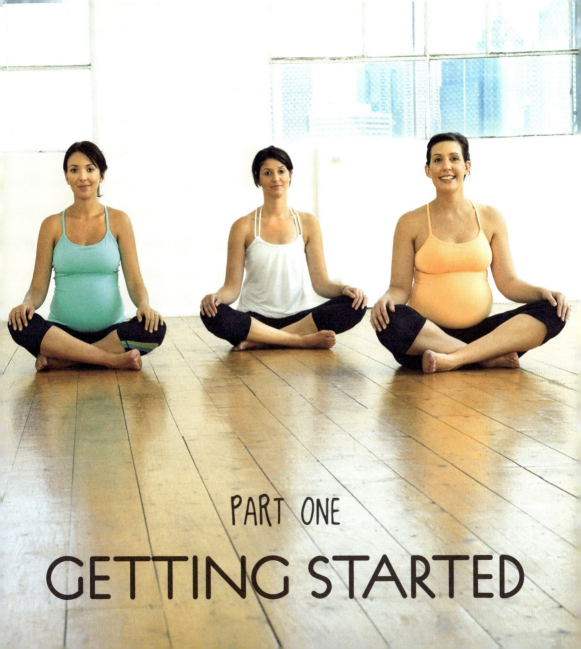

PART ONE
GETTING STARTED

How to use this book

Whether you are planning a family, are a friend or relative of a pregnant woman, a fitness instructor working with mums-to-be, or are pregnant yourself, *Exercising for Two* is designed to help women exercise safely during their pregnancy. Becoming aware of the changes in your body that go hand-in-hand with pregnancy helps you to understand why and how you need to modify your exercise program so you can safely enjoy the benefits of a prenatal fitness program.

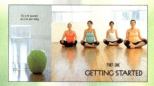

Outlines the general changes that happen to your body and their exercise implications, as well as certain pregnancy-related conditions that may occur and how you can further modify your program.

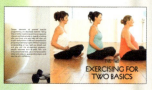

Hones in on the all-important pregnancy specifics that require extra thought and introduces you to exercise and pregnancy ground-rules.

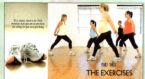

Every pregnancy is different so this section offers a comprehensive range of exercises, including those focused on mobility, sensible cardio training, strengthening, stretching, relaxing and practising for labour.

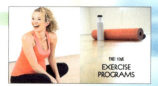

Fourteen prenatal exercise programs designed to help you choose the style and level of exercise that is just right for you and your baby.

you are unique

A certain move or workout can be ideal for one woman and completely inappropriate for another. One woman's warm-up is another woman's workout. Your fitness level, stage of pregnancy, general health and any pregnancy-related aches and pains all play a role in choosing the right style and level of exercise for you on any particular day. *Exercising for Two* outlines all the considerations of individual exercise selection and provides a range of options to help you customise your training, allowing you to confidently exercise according to your fitness, pregnancy, and specific needs. Remember, every day is a new day and things can change so always listen to your body.

Every woman is different, every pregnancy is unique

The benefits of prenatal exercise

Sensible exercise is imperative for a healthy pregnancy, delivery and baby

While there are some pregnancies where rest is more important than working out, most mums-to-be can enjoy a sensible exercise program safely – reaping a range of physical and psychological benefits for your health and well-being, fitness, comfort, labour preparation and postnatal recovery. Appropriate exercise during your pregnancy has the following benefits for both mother and baby.

Support a nine-month physical and psychological journey

Developing your fitness and strength will aid your stamina, posture and overall health throughout your pregnancy and labour. Participating in a carefully selected exercise program will also give you valuable time to yourself and help you manage the physical and emotional changes that go hand-in-hand with pregnancy and childbirth.

Maintain fitness and muscle tone

The right combination of exercises can help maintain cardiovascular fitness, strength and muscle tone. Honing in on specific areas, such as your posture, pelvic floor and core muscles is imperative.

Maintain a healthy body weight

It is natural and important to put on weight as your baby develops and sensible exercise and a nutritious diet will help you to stay within a healthy weight range throughout your pregnancy.

Keep your back in action
Specific mobility, core- and back-strengthening exercises will help you adjust to and accommodate the growing weight of your baby. As your pregnancy progresses, exercises that strengthen your back and enhance your awareness of the gradual postural changes will allow you to correct and support your carriage, avoiding common problems such as backache.

Sleep a little easier
Rest, relaxation and stretching are important ingredients in your overall well-being. Regular exercise will help you relax, improving your sleep patterns for a better night's sleep.

Boost your mood and self-esteem
Whether you choose to join other mums-to-be in a prenatal class, or enjoy a peaceful walk or workout alone, there is no doubt that exercise is a fabulous tonic to refresh and re-energise you.

Minimise aches and pains
Suitable exercise during pregnancy can protect against health issues such as constipation, incontinence, backache and pelvic joint pain, and with careful selection help you continue to exercise without aggravating existing conditions.

Prepare for labour
A healthy, strong body and a positive attitude are important factors to get you through the physical and psychological challenges during labour.

Get your body back in shape
A regular fitness routine will also help you to recover sooner and get back in shape more quickly after your little bundle has arrived.

Before You Start

Discussing your pregnancy exercise program with your health provider will give you a framework to work within. As your pregnancy progresses and your body changes you may need to adapt your exercise accordingly. Most women experience a low-risk pregnancy and are able to exercise within the guidelines suggested. Modifying your regular exercise program when you are expecting is important to avoid aches, pains and complications. A few modifications here and there will prevent stress on vulnerable joints and muscles, and protect against compromising your baby's development or your own comfort. Additional focus on areas such as pelvic floor, core, posture and back strength are particularly important for women in the childbearing years. But every pregnancy is different and some women need to modify their exercise regime more than others. Allowing your body to change and adapt as your baby develops and allowing your mind to accept, acknowledge and enjoy this special time are equally important. Your health situation can change over the course of nine months and it is important to have your health and pregnancy reviewed regularly. It is also important to tune into what is happening with your body. If something doesn't feel right, get yourself checked before you continue exercising.

There is no better time than now to commence your pregnancy wellness program.

Your pre-pregnancy overhaul

The following tips will help you and your baby thrive over the upcoming months.

- A little fitness under your belt will help prepare your body for pregnancy and motherhood.
- Avoid overdoing it – before or during pregnancy is a good time for balancing exercise, healthy habits and rest.
- Clean up your diet – include plenty of fresh vegetables and fruit, wholegrain cereals and sensible amounts of lean protein.
- Drink plenty of water and avoid caffeine and alcohol.
- Discuss with your healthcare provider your prescription and non-prescription medication – they will advise on the right vitamins and supplements to take (e.g. folic acid).
- Have any aches or pains assessed and treated by your physiotherapist or healthcare provider.
- Now is a great time to give up smoking.
- Make sleep, rest and relaxation a priority.

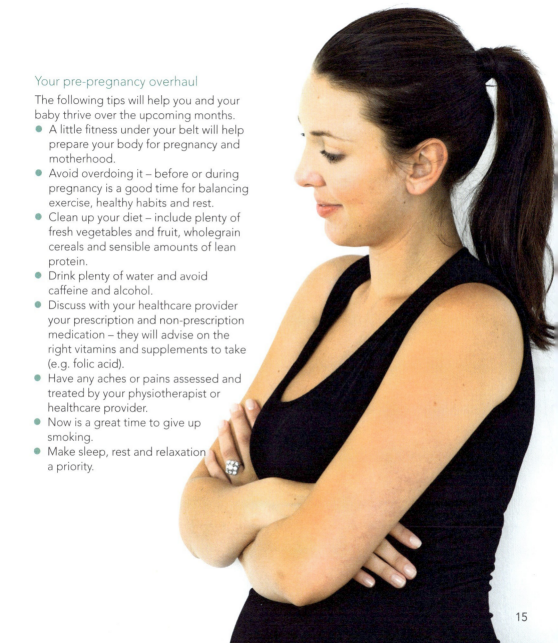

can exercise harm me and my baby?

No. If you have a healthy, low risk pregnancy exercise can be very beneficial for both mother and baby. The critical thing is to only undertake exercises that are safe and at the appropriate level for your individual situation, taking into account pre-existing fitness and stage of pregnancy. The right exercises can be an important ingredient in a safe and comfortable pregnancy, delivery and birth.

You can also benefit from attending a physiotherapy prenatal fitness class. As well as meeting other pregnant women, you will receive excellent instruction, supervision and exercises, custom-designed for pregnancy. A carefully planned fitness regime will allow you to continue activities that will assist, rather than exacerbate, your condition, aches or pains.

As a general rule, it is recommended that you avoid long periods of intense exercise, moves that jolt your joints and pelvic floor or positions and activities that may stress your body or compromise blood flow to the uterus. With a sound understanding of your pregnancy, what's happening with your body and its limitations, plus some old-fashioned common sense, you can select a program that suits your needs to reap the benefits of exercising as you and your baby grow together.

Know your body, listen to your body and enjoy the results

When rest is best

There are a few medical conditions that can develop during pregnancy, which mean you can only perform gentle activities such as pelvic floor lifts and circulation exercises. In the unlikely event you develop any of the following conditions, you will be advised to avoid exercise and rest. Your doctor will advise you of your specific needs;
● incompetent cervix ● intrauterine growth retardation ● maternal heart disease ● placenta praevia after 26 weeks ● pre-eclampsia ● restrictive lung disease ● uncontrolled hypertension ● venous or pulmonary thrombosis ● persistent bleeding ● preterm labour.

When you need to be especially careful

While it is still safe to exercise, some women experience pregnancy-related conditions that require extra supervision, advice and exercise modification. If you have any of the following conditions, consult your healthcare provider or physiotherapist for further advice and how to modify your exercise appropriately: ● pelvic joint pain ● back pain ● incontinence ● being significantly over- or underweight ● carpel tunnel syndrome ● gestational diabetes ● multiple pregnancy ● gastric reflux ● other aches and pains

Know when you need to stop

No matter what your fitness level, if you experience any of the following symptoms when exercising, you should stop activity immediately and contact your healthcare provider: ● abdominal cramps ● chest pain or palpitations ● dizziness or feeling faint ● excessive shortness of breath ● feeling unusually hot or overheated ● intense back pain ● nausea or vomiting ● ruptured membranes ● severe headache ● sudden joint pain ● sudden swelling in your hands, feet or ankles ● vaginal bleeding.

Why you need to modify your exercise

Alongside the wonderful creation and growth of a new little person, comes a variety of significant hormonal, physiological and psychological changes. These affect your ability to exercise safely, in a range of ways, some more than others. An awareness of the main changes and their exercise implications enables you to understand why and how you should modify your fitness program so that you can be confident you are making the right decisions for your body and your growing baby.

Cardiovascular changes + exercise implications

Just being pregnant is a workout. When you are pregnant, your heart and lungs work a little harder. Your blood volume, cardiac output, respiratory rate and resting heart rate increase. Your heart is pumping about one extra litre of blood around your body and your oxygen uptake rises. Alongside this your metabolism is also raised. In simple terms, your heart, lungs and metabolism respond to pregnancy like you are already exercising. When you consider the energy that goes into a developing baby, it is no wonder that a mum-to-be can feel a little tired. Acknowledging that being pregnant means your body is working harder is helpful. You may find you need to review your exercise intensity and how much you are trying to squeeze into your day. Most importantly, listen to your body. There might be times when putting your feet up is better for you and your baby than a workout. Try to find time to relax for a half hour every day. Your body and baby will thank you.

Hormones on the move + exercise implications

Three hormones, oestrogen, progesterone and relaxin, have a starring role in your pregnancy, responsible for all those changes in your body – breast changes, uterine growth and healthy weight gain – as well as for common 'side effects' such as nausea, indigestion, varicose veins, constipation and bleeding gums. These important changes are all preparing you and your body for labour, childbearing and breastfeeding. Certain pregnancy hormones are associated with unexpected mood swings and physical discomforts too. But remember that they are all working for the well-being of your growing baby. Relaxin, which accommodates your growing bump and sets you up for labour, is of specific relevance to exercise because it makes your joints more vulnerable. Produced in the early weeks of pregnancy, it continues to be present many months after delivery. Softening the connective tissue (collagen) in ligaments, relaxin makes them more elastic but less supportive to joint stability. Increased ligament laxity means joints are more susceptible to strain and injury. Those joints that take extra load, such as your lower back, pelvis, hips, knees and feet being particularly at risk. Relaxin also softens the walls of veins which, in conjunction with increased blood flow, leads to an increased chance of varicose veins. Compromised joint stability and the associated risk of injury is one of the main reasons that low-impact and non-contact activities are recommended over stressful, jolting or high-impact ones during pregnancy. This is also why you should avoid extreme load, range of motion and stretches and why postural awareness, core stability and movement control are imperative.

Weight gain + exercise implications

Healthy weight gain is natural and important as your baby grows. As well as the baby's development, the growth of your uterus, increased blood volume, and added breast tissue all contribute to the healthy 12 to 15 extra kilograms you will gain during your pregnancy. This varies from woman to woman according to their pre-pregnancy weight and, of course, diet and activity levels. While gaining excess body fat may be undesirable, it is natural to put on a little extra, especially around your hips. Just as squirrels store nuts for winter, your body is preparing for the high energy demands of breastfeeding. Rather than feeling concerned, rejoice in your changing shape. Welcoming the changes and having pride as your body grows allows a healthy, happy mindset and attitude to your pregnancy. Although weight gain is natural and important it has repercussions all the same; the extra load on your body places stress through your joints and the expansion of your mid-section threatens your posture and back health. A sensible exercise and nutrition plan will help you maintain healthy weight gain without too many unwanted extra kilos. Postural awareness plus specific core strengthening exercises will help keep your back healthy. Selecting low-impact, and non-jolting exercises and avoiding moves that overload your joints will assist in the prevention of unwanted joint strain and discomfort.

Your muscles + exercise implications

Your abdominals and pelvic floor muscles are stretched and weakened as your baby grows, but there is plenty you can do to look after these muscles to avoid any negative consequences of their changes. A general strengthening program is a great way to maintain your strength and muscle tone during pregnancy. Extra focus on muscles is especially important during pregnancy – avoiding stress and incorporating specific strengthening of your abdominals and pelvic floor – deserves high priority (pages 89–97).

The all-important pelvic floor + exercise implications

One in three mothers experiences incontinence. If every woman understood and prioritised the importance of looking after her pelvic floor during pregnancy this might not be the case. The pelvic floor is a group of muscles lying between your tail bone, pubic bone and sit bones. It supports your bowel, bladder and uterus and your growing baby. There are three passages that come down through the pelvic floor: the urethra, rectum and, in women, the vagina. A strong pelvic floor is vital for continence (bladder and bowel control) and helps to prevent prolapse (dropping down of the pelvic organs). It plays a significant role in the prevention of lower back pain as it is one of the spinal stabilising muscles. Also, a strong pelvic floor increases sensation during sex. Ideally, everyone would include the pelvic floor in their exercise regime – but, being a muscle that is out of sight it is also 'out of mind' and commonly neglected until symptoms occur. Pregnancy is certainly a time to prioritise your pelvic floor. It is inevitable that the pelvic floor bears extra load during pregnancy and childbirth; the added stress tends to stretch and weaken the muscles, compromising function. The main risk of a weakened pelvic floor is incontinence and prolapse. While it is not unusual for a woman to experience a little leakage when she moves suddenly, coughs or laughs, especially in the last trimester, or soon after delivery, this is not normal and you should not just accept it as part of motherhood and ignore it. There is plenty you can do to optimise your pelvic floor's integrity and function. Most importantly avoid compromising your pelvic floorwith stressful activities such as high impact exercise, heavy lifting and straining . While it is wise to give most muscle groups 'days off', when you're pregnant you should exercise your pelvic floor daily; three times per day for just a few minutes each time. Opt for quality not quantity and vary your training. Your pelvic floor needs to support your baby and pelvic contents all day, every day, as well as be able to switch on with a fast, strong contraction when you laugh and cough or move suddenly. You should cross-train your pelvic floor, sometimes including long holds for endurance and other times strong, quick lifts. Choose from the selection of pelvic floor options on pages 89–97 for a balanced daily pelvic-floor regime. As well as being able to lift your pelvic floor, being aware of how it feels to relax it is also important and especially useful in labour.

Your abdominals + exercise implications

It is no surprise that your abdominals must lengthen to accommodate your growing baby. This means the muscles are compromised in their ability to function, and less able to support your spine and pelvis. There are several reasons why you should alter your abdominal training during pregnancy. It is recommended that you cease all exercises lying on your back from 16 weeks onwards (see supine hypotension on page 25) but even early on abdominal curls should be minimised to avoid increasing your risk of Diastasis Rectus Abdominus (abdominal separation). Your abdominal muscles are united in the midline by a strong fibrous sheath (linea alba). The combination of pregnancy hormones and an expanding abdomen can lead to a widening and an area of separation, most commonly just above or below the navel. This diastasis compromises the mechanical efficiency and stabilising role of your abs, which means you are at higher risk of lower back pain. Certain factors increase the likelihood and degree of separation; weight gain, age, having a larger baby or twins, connective tissue insufficiencies and subsequent pregnancies. Overly toned, tight rectus muscles are more vulnerable to separation; and why excessive abdominal training is discouraged, even early in pregnancy (when the supine position is not yet a concern). To asses for a diastasis lie on your back with your knees slightly bent and your fingers aligned along your midline, above or below your navel. As you raise your head and shoulders you will feel a trough or raised ridge if a separation exists. If you detect a diastasis, seek advice from your physiotherapist or health care provider. Many traditional abdominal exercises (e.g. ab curls) that place stress on both the pelvic floor and the outer abdominals, are best avoided. The core stabilising role of your abs however has never been more important. Accept that your abdominals must lengthen, do not try to keep them tight and strong by doing sit ups, curls and hovers. The chance of separation, plus the need to avoid supine exercises means you should replace these moves with sensible prenatal options such as core stability training (see pages 100–115) whilst sitting or in four point kneeling.

Your circulation + exercise implications

As your baby grows, lying on your back to exercise is not recommended. The reason: the weight of your growing uterus – after 16 weeks' gestation or more – may compress major blood vessels and possibly affect your blood pressure and the blood-flow to the placenta. This is known as supine hypotension. Do not worry if you naturally sleep on your back, this is very different to exercising, but if you prefer you can put a pillow under your hip and shoulder so you are slightly off your back. You may hear conflicting opinions such as, 'It's fine to exercise on your back until the mother feels light-headed', but it is the possible compromised blood-flow to the placenta that leads me to caution you; if in doubt, leave it out. One of the most popular supine exercises is the abdominal curl; you should avoid these during pregnancy (see pages 56–57 for more information). Don't despair, there are plenty of excellent alternatives to supine exercises on offer that provide a safe, effective and comprehensive workout. A heavy uterus in later stages of pregnancy can also compromise blood-flow back from your legs to your heart, when you are standing still, making you feel light-headed. This is also due to the fact that your veins are altered by pregnancy hormones that make them more dilated. By moving your legs your muscles help to pump the blood up your veins and thus avoid the faint feeling associated with standing hypotension. Choose from a range of excellent alternatives to supine exercises. Remember, in the big picture it's a short time. Avoid prolonged stationary standing (standing still), especially after activities such as cycling or walking, which divert extra blood-flow to your legs. Walking on the spot between standing strength exercises or sitting down on a fitball to perform upper body exercises will also help prevent standing hypotension. Specifically designed pressure support stockings made for pregnant women may help prevent symptoms of standing hypotension and varicose veins. Calf raises or walking on the spot might help if you feel these symptoms in situations such as standing at the supermarket.

Your core temperature + exercise implications

It is important to avoid overheating, especially during the first trimester, when your baby's major organs are developing. A pregnant woman's core temperature is naturally slightly raised and whilst we know exercise is beneficial, working out to the point of feeling hot, sweaty and extremely short of breath is not recommended. This is one of the main reasons to modify your training, especially your cardiovascular exercise, even before you look pregnant. Your ideal activity level is mild to moderate, rather than intense. A fit person can work harder than a sedentary person without overheating so it stands to reason that your training level depends on your pre-existing fitness. Raised core temperature is related to both how hard you work and for how long, thus gentle activity can be performed safely for longer than more energetic exercise. You should feel like you are exercising but be able to talk during your workout and not be exhausted. Taking your heart rate is one way to assess your workout level. Traditional guidelines recommend you should not train at heart rates over 140–150 beats per minute. Perceived exertion is another guide to safe exercise intensity: On a scale of 1 to 20 with 1 being at rest and 20 being highly energetic, aim to work at an intensity of 12 to 13. (See pages 60–61 for important tips on how to gauge intensity and avoid overheating).

Your joints + exercise implications
Weight gain, pregnancy hormones and altered posture mean your joints are more vulnerable during pregnancy. This is another reason to keep your exercise low impact, smooth and controlled. Take extra care to avoid undue stress on your joints, especially those particularly at risk, which include those of the pelvis, lower back, feet, wrists and thoracic spine. (See pages 30–35). Checking for good posture and avoiding extreme load or range of movement helps you protect your joints as you maintain your prenatal fitness plan.

Your digestion + exercise implications
The hormones of pregnancy can play games with your digestive system, slowing down your gut activity and digestion, allowing longer for nutritional absorption (which is a good thing) but also causing a tendency for constipation, indigestion, heartburn and reflux. The latter may be increased as the growth of your baby pushes on your stomach. Eating healthy, small meals more often will help prevent the discomfort of heartburn. Avoid exercising after eating. Making sure you drink plenty of water and a healthy high-fibre diet full of fruit, vegies and complex carbohydrates will help prevent constipation; exercise can also lend a hand. If you experience reflux or indigestion you are likely to prefer upright positions such as standing or sitting, to horizontal positions, such as side-lying or kneeling on all fours.

Eat, drink and exercise

Your pelvic ligaments + exercise implications

The round and the broad ligaments support the uterus within the pelvis. As your baby grows you may notice a sudden sharp or 'pulling' sensation in your groin or lower back area associated with movement, for example when standing up quickly. This discomfort is brief but disconcerting. It is not affected by exercise but may serve as a reminder to avoid sudden or jerky movements. If you experience any new or ongoing discomfort, however, you should stop exercising and seek advice from your healthcare professional.

Your bladder + exercise implications

It is quite normal to need to go to the bathroom more often when you are expecting. Early on, this is due to hormonal and cardiovascular changes and later it is due to your growing bub and uterus pressing on your bladder. It is very important that you maintain healthy hydration by drinking plenty of water, and simply accept that you will need to go more often. Ideally, there will be a bathroom near to where you exercise. If you need to go to the bathroom during your workout always get up slowly and avoid rushing. This is especially important if you are getting out of the pool.

Your breasts + exercise implications

As your pregnancy progresses your breasts will change. Always wear a comfortable, supportive maternity bra that is free of restrictive underwire and check your upper body posture remains tall and slouch-free. Breast comfort is yet another reason to avoid high-impact or bouncy movements.

Carrying twins + exercise implications

While exercise programs during an uncomplicated twin pregnancy may follow similar guidelines to a single pregnancy, it is important to recognise the increased risks and areas for special care. Extra medical supervision and guidance is recommended. If you are expecting twins and feeling fine, you can enjoy a sensible exercise program. Your body is doing an important job so keep in mind you are more likely to feel tired and more prone to certain aches, pains and conditions. Listen to your body, get plenty of rest and exercise under the guidance of your pregnancy care provider.

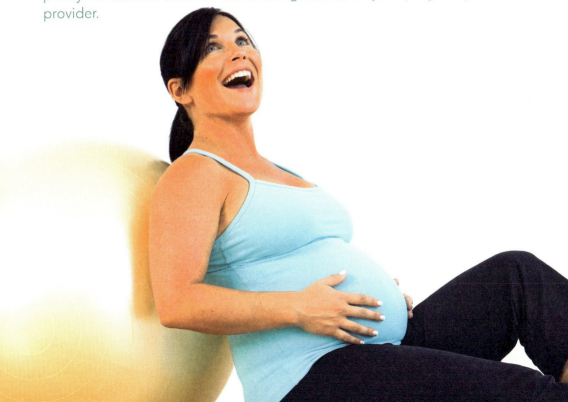

When you need to take extra care and modify your exercise further

There are a few conditions that can occur during pregnancy, requiring extra care and modifications where exercise is concerned. The wrong exercise may aggravate the issues, but the good news is that if you understand your situation and modify accordingly, you can continue to exercise safely. In fact, specific exercises can help you manage or alleviate the condition.

Morning sickness + exercise implications

The hormones that help to sustain pregnancy can also cause nausea and vomiting, commonly referred to as morning sickness. Women who experience mild nausea often find that exercise relieves their symptoms, others however experience more extreme symptoms, which limit their ability to exercise, eat and drink and may require medical assistance. While you should not exercise on a full stomach, it is also important you have had a healthy snack or meal within the last few hours to avoid hypoglycaemia (low blood sugar). Therefore, if you are unable to eat breakfast, for example, you may have to train in the afternoons. Mums-to-be sometimes feel too unwell or tired to exercise initially and so don't commence exercise until after the first trimester. If this is the case, it's important to remember that even if you were active prior to your pregnancy you've now had 12 weeks off, so start back slowly and progress gradually.

Adjust your program to suit

Indigestion and reflux + exercise implications
Indigestion and reflux (or heartburn) are more likely when you're expecting due to a combination of hormonal effects, delayed gastric emptying, your oesophageal sphincter being less efficient and the fact that your uterus causes pressure on your stomach as your baby grows. Eat smaller and more frequent meals and avoid exercising immediately after eating. Avoid bouncy exercise styles. Find alternatives to horizontal positions such as recumbent side-lying, kneeling or sitting.

Fluid and swelling + exercise implications
It is not unusual to notice a little swelling in your feet, ankles and fingers, especially later in your pregnancy. Avoid tight clothing and try to put your feet up each day. Exercise helps boost blood flow and circulation, which can help decrease swelling. Aqua exercise is particularly helpful as the hydrostatic pressure of the water helps to move the fluid out of the tissues back into the circulating blood system, as does wearing pregnancy-specific pressure stockings. If swelling increases or you feel unwell, consult your healthcare provider as soon as possible.

Get some support and put your feet up

Pelvic-joint pain + exercise
The bones of your pelvis join together like a bowl, its base being the pelvic floor. It has one joint at the front (the pubic symphysis) and two joints at the back, either side of the triangular-shaped sacrum (the sacroiliac joints). You may experience inflammation and pain in these joints due to the extra load of your growing baby, and hormonal-induced ligament and joint laxity.

Symptoms range from slight discomfort to extreme pain with compromised function and difficulty walking. Pelvic joint pain can also cause referred pain into your buttock or down the back of your thigh. It is important to differentiate it from lower back pain as the exercise implications differ for the two. There is increased risk with subsequent pregnancies. The most common causes of pregnancy-related pelvic joint pain, also known as 'pelvic instability' include: asymmetrical weight-bearing (taking weight through one leg more than the other), e.g. standing while holding your toddler on one hip ● repetitive weight shift from one foot to the other, e.g. taking long walks or using stairs ● long periods of standing ● wide stance, e.g. doing a wide squat ● uneven wide stance or weight-shift, e.g. alternating lunges ● rotation, e.g. swivelling to get out of the car ● muscle imbalances ● lack of core strength. Unfortunately, for those who experience pelvic joint pain, walking is not recommended, as the shift of weight from foot to foot is aggravating. This can be frustrating if you have been enjoying long walks, especially if you have a dog. Walking up stairs or training on a step is even worse. Standing or kneeling on one leg, whilst exercising the other, will also cause or exacerbate the pain as will alternating lunges, rotating your pelvis or wide squats. The good news is that there are plenty of great alternatives. Exercises that take the load and stress off the pelvis are ideal, such as sitting on a fitball and aqua exercise. Swimming is great because of the relieving effect of buoyancy but the kicking part of breaststroke should be avoided. If you have pelvic joint discomfort a helpful attitude is to exercise and perform daily activities as though you are wearing a miniskirt. Narrow base squats are better than wide ones, getting out of the car or up off the floor with your knees together is less aggravating than moving one leg after the other. It is also important to work on core stabilising exercises and specific stretches of the deep posterior hip muscles, which help some people but not everyone. See pages 100–115, 192. If you have pregnancy-related pelvic-joint pain you can continue to perform activities and exercises that do not aggravate the condition, but avoid moves that are stressful. In *Exercising for Two* the exercise repertoire specifically excludes any moves that stress the pelvic joints in order to avoid causing pelvic joint pain or instability.

Other joint discomforts
The load and laxity effects of pregnancy can also influence other joints, including those in your thoracic spine, lower back and feet:

Thoracic spine + exercise implications
The expanding effect of your rib cage to accommodate your growing baby in the final trimester leads to movement at the costo-vertebral joints, where your ribs meet your thoracic vertebrae. This can cause discomfort in your middle back or referred pain that spreads around the side of your rib cage. Exercise within comfort. You may find that seated rotation (see page 114) helps relieve the discomfort. Manual physiotherapy techniques may also help.

Lower back pain + exercise implications
A common condition during pregnancy due to altered posture and extra load. Avoid the temptation to stand with a swayed back and make good posture your priority (see pages 98–99). Avoid positions and activities that strain your back, such as abdominal curls, push-ups or heavy lifting, and include plenty of sensible back and core stability strengthening. Kneeling on all fours, using a fitball and water-based exercises are all great options for your back. See your physiotherapist for assessment and management if you experience new or ongoing back pain.

Feet + exercise implications

Many women find they go up about half a shoe size during pregnancy (quite annoying if your favourite shoes no longer fit!). This is due to a small drop in the arch of your foot in response to laxity and added load. Supportive footwear has never been more important. Avoid activities that cause your feet to hurt and check you do not curl your toes or try to grip with your feet when standing and exercising. Use this as a good excuse for a foot massage!

Carpal tunnel syndrome + exercise implications

The nerves and blood vessels that supply your hands pass through a confined space across your wrists known as the carpal tunnel. Oedema or swelling can lead to compression of the nerves and vessels causing discomfort, altered sensation, pins and needles or weakness in your hands. If you have carpal tunnel syndrome you should avoid weight-bearing through your wrists. If your ability to grip is compromised it is unwise to use hand weights. Immersing your wrists and hands alternately in warm and cold water and gentle wrist mobility exercises may assist circulation and thus decrease oedema. You should also speak with your doctor or physiotherapist regarding the option of wrist splints.

Varicose veins and vulval varicosities + exercise implications

Pregnancy hormones, extra blood volume and compromised venous return when you are standing combine to make you more prone to varicose veins in your legs. Increased discomfort is caused by blood pooling associated with stationary standing (standing still). Vulval varicosities are in an awkward area and can make sitting uncomfortable. Avoid prolonged standing whenever possible. Use muscle pump activity to assist circulation.

For example, walk rather than stand still. Wear pregnancy-specific support stockings or tights and avoid tight clothing, especially socks. Put your feet and legs up on the couch as much as possible. Aqua exercise is a great option as hydrostatic pressure assists circulation. Wear firm and supportive underpants to provide some relief for vulval varicosities.

Diabetes + exercise implications

If you have diabetes before you became pregnant or you develop gestational diabetes during your pregnancy it is important to check your blood sugar levels regularly plus seek nutritional and exercise advice to manage this condition. If your blood glucose is well-controlled you should be able to continue to exercise. In fact, exercise can be beneficial in the control of diabetes.

Haemorrhoids + exercise implications

Hormones and pressure increase the chance of haemorrhoids during pregnancy. Constipation only adds to the problem. A healthy diet, drinking plenty of water and taking your time on the toilet are all important. See your healthcare provider for specific advice. Avoid stationary standing and it may also be necessary to find alternatives to sitting. Include plenty of water, fibre and fresh fruit and vegetables in your diet and do not rush when using the toilet. Ice-packs may help and if it is a significant problem you should speak to a women's health physiotherapist about defecation techniques to avoid exacerbating the symptoms.

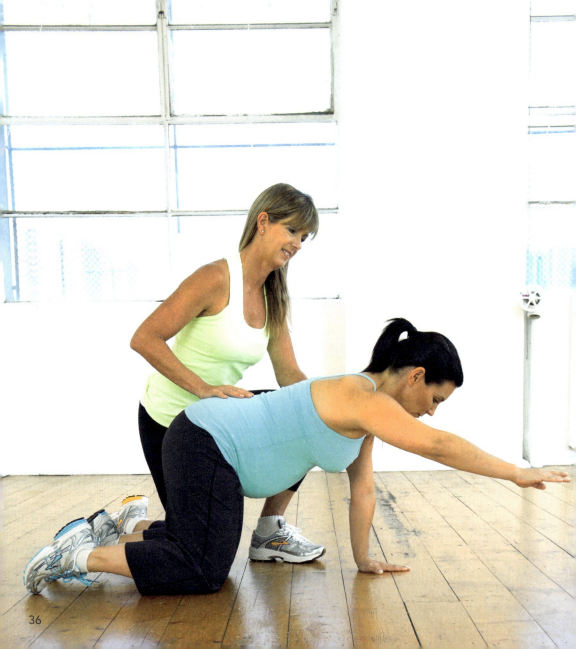

Choose exercises that suit you and your baby

Whilst safety is imperative, it is also important to discover exercise styles that you enjoy and a program that suits your lifestyle. Aqua exercise, for example, is a great choice during pregnancy, but if you dislike getting your hair wet, or you don't have access to a pool, a water-based exercise program is not for you. Varying your routine is ideal; it keeps your interest high and the stresses on your body low. *Exercising for Two* delivers a range of exercise styles and programs for everyone, allowing you to explore, enjoy and reap the benefits of a varied and interesting pregnancy fitness program. There are also a number of options to help you discover an exercise style that will suit you and your lifestyle.

Group exercise classes

Visit any health and fitness club and you are sure to find a diverse selection of group exercise classes on offer. Group exercise classes are fun, motivational and social, although not all classes are appropriate for mums-to-be. Ideally, you will attend a class that is specifically for pregnant women, run by a person who is well-qualified to design and instruct a prenatal fitness program. If you have been attending fitness classes prior to pregnancy, and you are feeling fit and well, you may choose to continue, but you would be wise to select classes that are low impact and allow you to work at a moderate intensity. Aqua aerobics, pilates and fitball classes are more likely to suit your body's changing needs. Always watch or try a class before committing to regular attendance. Check your instructor is well-qualified to understand and provide alternatives to your specific needs and that the class content is safe and sensible for pregnancy.

Avoid classes that:
- are high impact, high energy or otherwise inappropriate
- include overload on your abdominals or pelvic floor
- are stressful on your joints, especially your back and pelvis
- devote significant time to inappropriate positions, e.g. lying on your back.

General fitness class guidelines
- Advise the instructor you're pregnant and will be modifying accordingly.
- Ideally, attend a physiotherapy-led pregnancy-specific exercise class.
- Modify your workout intensity to moderate or a perceived exertion of 13 (see pages 60–61).
- Take frequent rests and keep your cardiovascular component to 30 minutes or less.
- Replace high-impact exercise with controlled low-impact exercise.
- Avoid complex moves, sudden changes in direction and twisting.
- Replace exercises that significantly work your outer abdominals with inner-core stability options, such as sitting on a ball or in four-point kneeling.
- Avoid exercising lying on your back.
- Avoid exercises that place undue stress on your pelvic joints, such as wide-based squats, grapevines, side steps, lunges and those that weight-bear through one leg more than the other.
- If in doubt, replace an exercise with pelvic floor or core training.

Fitness-class styles

High/low aerobics

These high energy, high-impact classes are fun but not the ideal option for you and your baby. Due to the heating factor of these classes, the impact on joints and, most importantly, the bouncing and load on your pelvic floor, low-impact classes are a preferable choice.

Low-impact aerobics

These classes are still energetic, but less stressful on your joints and pelvic floor. Focus on keeping your core and pelvic floor engaged and avoid bouncing movements, instead taking your pelvis and your baby for a smooth ride. Steer away also from wide-based stepping actions, twisting movements and any exercise that strains your joints, back or abdominals. Low-impact classes are inappropriate for women with pelvic joint or lower back discomfort.

Step classes

Step classes, although 'low impact', are high energy so a poor choice for anyone new to exercise, even in the first trimester. If you are used to step classes and wish to continue you should lower your platform and focus on smooth, controlled low-impact movement, maintaining core and pelvic-floor recruitment and moderate intensity. It is important to note that stepping up and down on a platform is stressful to your pelvic joints so anyone worried they might experience pelvic joint pain should not perform step aerobics and certainly stop doing them if they experience even a hint of discomfort.

Cycling classes
Indoor cycling classes are a popular cardiovascular fitness option. They are extremely energetic, motivating and usually run for 45 minutes or longer. This is too long and too energetic for anyone but the very fittest pregnant women. I would encourage all pregnant women to consider alternatives such as fitball or aqua fitness. If you wish to continue cycling now that you are pregnant it is vital you lower your resistance so that you maintain moderate intensity. Taking frequent rests and sipping water throughout will help prevent overheating (see pages 60–61). Focus on keeping your back straight and maintaining core recruitment. Most cycling classes involve music tracks where you are encouraged to turn up the resistance, stand up and push hard through your legs, as though climbing a hill; this places too much strain through your pelvis. During these tracks you should lighten your resistance and cycle gently, taking the opportunity to rest.

Combat classes
Martial arts-based combat classes are intense and involve high-impact jogging plus kicking and punching movements. These actions are stressful on your joints, especially your pelvic joints, and compromise your pelvic floor.

Circuit training
Circuit training classes involve performing various exercises as you go from station to station. Their content varies so much that one class may be fine for pregnancy and another completely inappropriate. Ideally, you would go to a physiotherapy-designed, pregnancy-specific circuit class. Adhere to all the usual rules of intensity and modify movements that strain your joints, back or pelvic floor.

Fitball, aqua aerobics, pilates and yoga classes
These classes, in general, are fabulous pregnancy choices. They are low impact and have added focus on core, posture, breathing and pelvic floor. As with all general fitness classes, however, there are moves in these classes that should not be included during pregnancy. Avoid bouncing or jolting, supine exercises and strength moves that strain your abdominals, back or joints. Pregnancy-specific fitball, aqua, pilates or yoga classes are ideal during this precious time.

Working out at the gym

If you have been working out in the gym prior to pregnancy you may choose to continue but modify to suit. Listen to your body. It is important to have your gym program assessed and modified by a women's health physiotherapist or fitness trainer with significant pregnancy-programming experience. Bring your cardio training back to moderate, low-impact levels and you may need to decrease your weights or resistance levels. If you are new to the gym you should seek programming advice from a physiotherapist or trainer with prenatal fitness knowledge and experience. Start with uncomplicated and sound options and build up gradually. Sensible equipment options for prenatal fitness include:

Treadmills
Walking rather than running is preferable for your joints and pelvic floor. If you are very fit and comfortable walking, add incline rather than speed. Intensity should range from a slow to a brisk walk for 5 to 30 minutes, depending on your fitness. Walking on treadmills is inappropriate if you have pelvic-joint pain.

Cycling

Cycling on stationary or recumbent bikes provides another low-impact cardiovascular training option. Keep the level low and avoid turning up the resistance to the point that requires you to push hard through one leg then the other. Maintain levels that allow you to stay seated and cycle comfortably. Exercising for 5 to 30 minutes at moderate intensity is ideal.

Strength and conditioning

The exercises described in this book can be performed in the gym or home. Free weights are an excellent option as long as you focus on fine form and technique. Make sure you maintain core control and smooth movement and are able to breathe throughout any strength move. Opt for sitting on a bench or fitball rather than standing whilst performing upper-body strengthening. Select narrow-based squats rather than lunges or wide squats. Focus on core training rather than outer-abdominal options. If you are confident using resistance machines you can continue, making sure you focus on your form and avoid inappropriate positions and load.

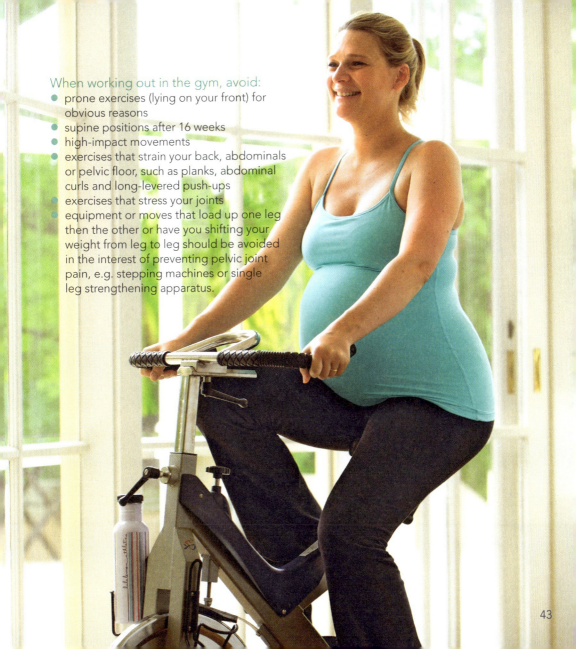

When working out in the gym, avoid:
- prone exercises (lying on your front) for obvious reasons
- supine positions after 16 weeks
- high-impact movements
- exercises that strain your back, abdominals or pelvic floor, such as planks, abdominal curls and long-levered push-ups
- exercises that stress your joints
- equipment or moves that load up one leg then the other or have you shifting your weight from leg to leg should be avoided in the interest of preventing pelvic joint pain, e.g. stepping machines or single leg strengthening apparatus.

Nutrition

Your basal metabolic rate increases during pregnancy to provide energy for your growing baby, placenta and uterus. If you are a healthy weight and maintaining sensible pregnancy activity and exercise levels, you will require on average an extra 850 to 1100 kJ per day.

A healthy diet, including a balance of all food groups, will help you optimise your well-being. Lean protein, plenty of fresh salad, fruit and vegetables and complex carbohydrates, such as whole grains and legumes are all recommended. Alcohol is best avoided and caffeine should be kept to one or two cups per day. Hydration is also important and whilst herbal teas and juices are fine, you really can't go past drinking plenty of good old H_2O.

During pregnancy there can be an increased need for certain nutrients, including protein, calcium, thiamine, folate, iodine and iron. Focusing on a healthy, varied diet before and during your pregnancy will help to meet these needs, but it is wise to discuss the possible need for supplementation with your doctor, in particular folate, which helps to reduce the risk of neural tube defects. Iron and iodine may also be recommended. If you have any questions or concerns about your prenatal nutrition, see a qualified dietitian.

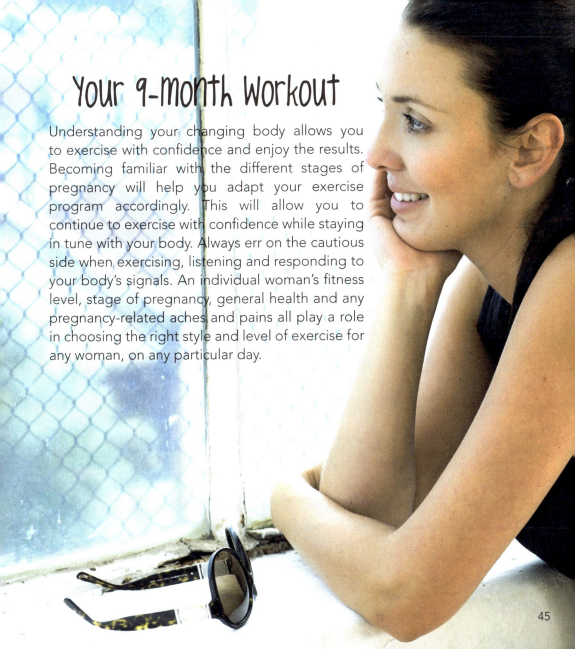

Your 9-month Workout

Understanding your changing body allows you to exercise with confidence and enjoy the results. Becoming familiar with the different stages of pregnancy will help you adapt your exercise program accordingly. This will allow you to continue to exercise with confidence while staying in tune with your body. Always err on the cautious side when exercising, listening and responding to your body's signals. An individual woman's fitness level, stage of pregnancy, general health and any pregnancy-related aches and pains all play a role in choosing the right style and level of exercise for any woman, on any particular day.

Certain elements of prenatal exercise programming are absolutely essential. Taking time to further explore issues that are especially relevant and high priority in regards to looking after your body and your baby will allow you to plan and practise a safe and comprehensive pregnancy exercise program. With an increased understanding of how hard you should work and why, and the all-important pregnancy-specific exercises, such as pelvic floor, core and postural exercises, you are empowered to select and enjoy an appropriate program and exercise with confidence.

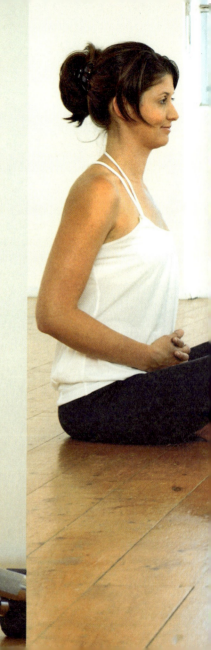

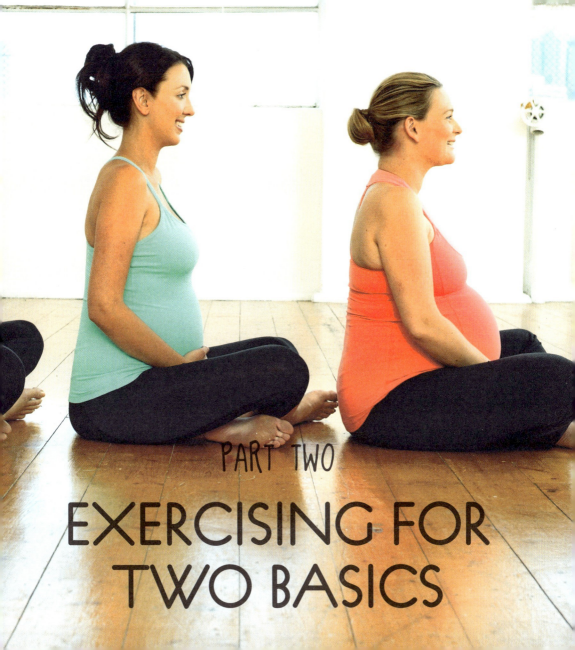

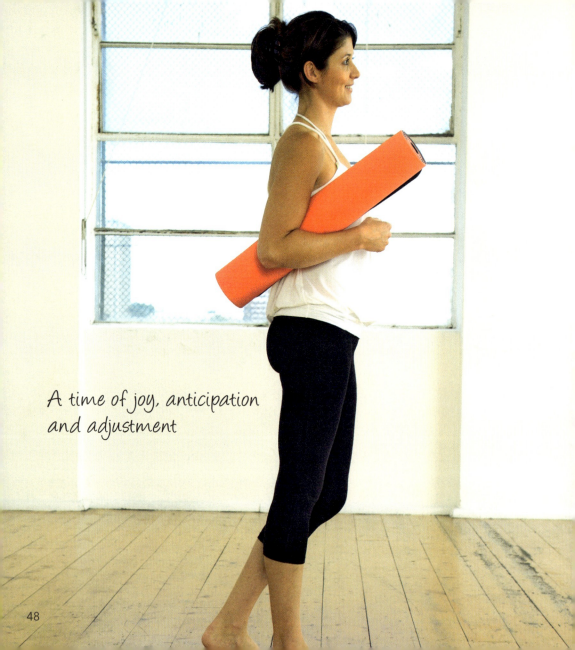

A time of joy, anticipation and adjustment

0 to 12 weeks
Exercising in the first trimester

While you may not yet look pregnant, your baby is very busy; this early stage is an important time for major foetal organ development, during which it is important you avoid overheating. This is why you should modify your exercise from the very beginning by keeping your exercising at a mild to moderate level, avoiding intensive exercise. As the weeks go by, the risk of miscarriage gradually decreases. If you have no prior history or risk of miscarriage you will be able to enjoy sensible exercise during the first trimester. If you are at an increased risk of miscarriage, you should avoid exercise until your healthcare provider gives you the all clear, usually in the second trimester. Women who have been inactive prior to pregnancy, but are otherwise well, should still take it easy, starting with very gentle exercises. In these early months it is important to take the time to enjoy your pregnancy and listen to your body; there may be times when rest is best.

First trimester basics
- Avoid exercise if there is identified risk or past history of miscarriage.
- Continue modified exercise if you have been exercising before becoming pregnant within the guidelines of this book.
- Prevent your body from overheating by keeping exercise at a moderate intensity and avoiding feeling hot, short of breath, sweaty or exhausted. See pages 60–61.
- Get started on pelvic floor, posture and core stability exercises.
- Choose low-impact exercise to minimise stress on vulnerable joints and your pelvic floor.
- Achieve a balance with work, exercise and rest.
- There has never been a better time to listen to your body.

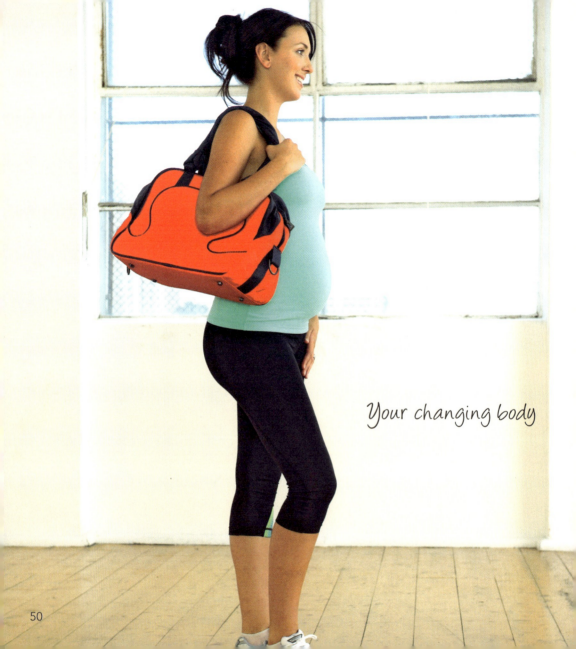

Your changing body

12 to 28 weeks
Exercising in the second trimester

During the second trimester you will notice your body changing and your abdomen expanding. With this comes altered posture, lengthened abdominal muscles and increased load on your pelvic floor and joints, especially those below the waist. Some women notice associated discomforts such as lower back pain or gastric reflux, all of which need to be accommodated in your exercise plan and daily activities. You may feel more energised now but it is still important to keep your exercise at a sensible level, ensuring it is smooth and low impact in the interest of looking after your baby, joints and pelvic floor. From 16 weeks onwards you should discontinue exercising on your back. It is also at around 16 weeks when you may notice small butterfly-like flutters, the first sensations of your baby moving.

Second trimester basics
- Continue pregnancy-appropriate exercise that suits your changing shape and situation.
- Mix low-impact fitness and strength training with pregnancy specifics, such as pelvic floor and core strengthening.
- Pay particular attention to correcting and strengthening your posture.
- Avoid supine (lying on your back) exercise from 16 weeks onwards.
- Avoid prolonged stationary standing.
- Be sure to have any new concern assessed by your healthcare provider and modify your exercise accordingly.

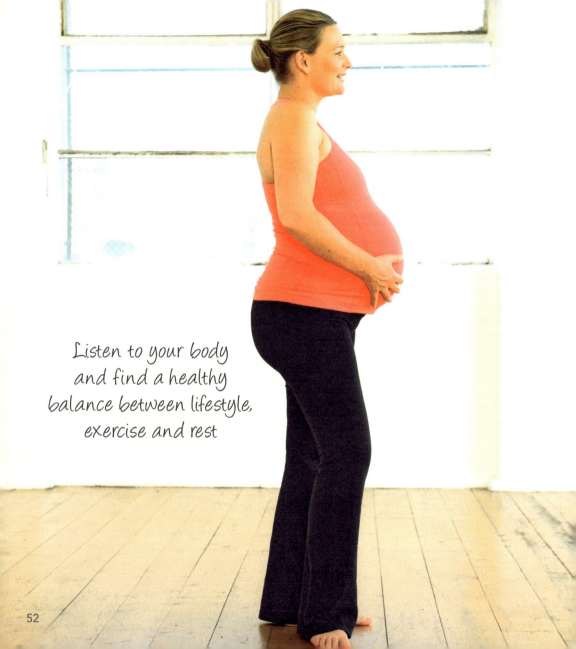

Listen to your body and find a healthy balance between lifestyle, exercise and rest

28 to 40 weeks
Exercising in the third trimester

It is no surprise that some women feel tired during these final months. As your baby grows and their organs mature during this time, your body will change even more, placing extra demand on your joints, posture and pelvic floor. With the extra space that your growing baby is taking up you might notice you are more prone to shortness of breath. But as baby moves downwards in preparation for delivery, you may experience relief in your breathing and a new heaviness in your pelvis. Exercise is still important now but you must select your options carefully to avoid aggravating or causing aches and pains. If you are having baby number two or three, looking after your toddler may be keeping you active enough. Putting your feet up on the couch and practising relaxation techniques in preparation for labour could also be more beneficial than going to the gym.

Third trimester basics
- Continue with moderate exercise, but within your comfort range.
- If you feel well, you can continue to exercise throughout your pregnancy.
- Concentrate on your core and pelvic floor.
- Avoid stressing your back or pelvis and try positions that take the load off these areas, e.g. kneeling on all fours.
- Continue to monitor your body and adapt your exercise for changes.
- If you have any concerns, seek professional advice.
- Labour preparation exercises and relaxation are valuable additions to your fitness program now. (See pages 180–87, 195–198.)

Pregnancy fitness fundamentals

There are four cornerstones that underpin safe, appropriate and effective fitness training during pregnancy that deserve extra thought and consideration.
1. Your pelvic floor fitness.
2. Your abdominal and core strengthening.
3. Your posture and back health.
4. Safe exercise intensity.

Your pelvic floor — an investment in the future

If there is one muscle group you must focus on and exercise daily when you're expecting, this is it. This muscular floor that supports your bladder, bowel and growing baby is vital for maintaining bladder and bowel control and also plays an important role in spinal stability and back health. It can be weakened by the load of your growing baby so it is vital that you avoid anything that adds stress to the pelvic floor and perform daily exercises to optimise its strength and function. Doing your pelvic floor exercises is vital (see pages 89–97), as is perfecting your technique.

There are several ways you can help maintain healthy pelvic floor function to assist the prevention of short- and long-term incontinence, prolapse and back pain. Basically, you must avoid exercises and activities that stress your pelvic floor and include exercises that strengthen it. If you have any concerns about your pelvic floor you should seek advice from a women's health and continence physiotherapist or speak to your doctor.

What can compromise pelvic floor strength and function?
● Pregnancy and childbirth ● straining due to constipation ● chronic coughing ● heavy lifting ● age ● obesity ● genetics ● high-impact exercise ● certain exercises such as wide squats, push-ups and abdominal curls ● chronic back pain.

Why should I keep my pelvic floor strong?
● Combat the weakening effect of pregnancy and childbirth ● Assist in the prevention of prolapse and incontinence, enhancing bladder and bowel control ● Help stabilise your spine and prevent lower back pain ● A strong pelvic floor improves sexual function and sensation ● Good pelvic floor awareness will also help you relax your pelvic floor during labour.

Exercising your pelvic floor basics:
- Exercise your pelvic floor 3–4 times per day.
- Technique matters – practise quality not quantity.
- Continue to breathe when lifting your pelvic floor.
- Avoid tensing other, unwanted muscle groups.
- Cross-train your pelvic floor; slow long holds for endurance, and strong fast lifts for strength.
- When exercising take your pelvis and your pelvic floor for a smooth ride, avoiding bouncing, jerking and jolting.
- Always recruit your pelvic floor before lifting or exercising.
- Put your feet up for at least 30 minutes per day.
- It is also important to become aware of how it feels to relax your pelvic floor.

Your abdominal muscles – the ins and outs

Abdominal exercises are important during pregnancy for supporting your spine, pelvis and baby but which ones are appropriate? It is the deep abdominal muscles that you cannot see, which are important during pregnancy, rather than the outer ones, commonly used for abdominal curls and sit-ups. Your abdominal muscles are arranged in layers; the outer layer is called rectus abdominis, followed by external obliques, internal obliques and – the deepest abdominal layer – the transverses abdominis. Each plays a different role, the outer layers being responsible for moving your torso by flexing and rotating the spine, and the deepest layers playing an important role in core stability, supporting your spine and pelvis. The spinal stabilising muscles are the ones that deserve your focus now, and there are several reasons why you should leave sit-ups and other strong outer abdominal exercises alone.

This is not the time for the six-pack

Five reasons to modify abdominal training:
1. Focusing on strong outer abdominals, even early on in pregnancy may increase risk of rectus abdominis separation.
2. You should not exercise lying on your back after 16 weeks.
3. Your abs don't work as they did pre-pregnancy.
4. Many outer abdominal muscle exercises strain your back and pelvic floor, which are already vulnerable.
5. Your core stabilising muscles are important for support of your spine, pelvis and pregnancy. These should be your abdominal focus.

Exercise basics for your abdominal muscles:
- Strong deep abdominals help support your spine, pelvis and pregnancy, but outer abdominals should not be put under stress or strain.
- Avoid excessive outer abdominal training, even early.
- Abdominal curls are inappropriate after 16 weeks.
- Core muscle focus is important and beneficial throughout pregnancy and after delivery.
- Core abdominals work with the pelvic floor and deep back muscles to help prevent incontinence and back pain.
- Modified outer abdominal exercises are included to help them maintain function and to assist postnatal recovery.
- Excellent abdominal alternatives include four-point kneel, sitting on fitball and numerous core exercises (see pages 100–115).
- Maintaining inner and outer abdominal integrity will help you get your body back in shape after you've delivered your baby.

Core stability – strong foundations

Core stability is one of the most important focuses of prenatal fitness. The deepest abdominal layer, transversus abdominus works with deep back muscles (multifidus) plus the pelvic floor below and diaphragm above create a cylinder that supports your lumbar spine. These stabilising muscles assist good posture, healthy movement and the prevention of back pain, all of which are even more important during pregnancy.

Strengthen your core

Deep stabilising muscles work together to support the spine. Training them correctly allows you to prevent or manage back pain and other discomforts such as pelvic instability. The focus is on gently drawing your lower abdomen inwards towards your lower back. You may notice a lifting of your pelvic floor, which is a good thing. Avoid the temptation of sucking in your ribs, bracing your tummy or holding your breath as these compromise core muscle function. When starting out perform very simple core exercises (see pages 100–111) and work your way up to more complex core conditioning exercise; (see pages 112–115). Always train for quality not quantity. Signs of over-challenging your core include shaky movement, holding your breath, tensing other muscles, clenching your fists, or shrugging your shoulders. If you feel this, decrease the intensity or core challenge of the exercise.

Core exercise basics:

- Place core and pelvic floor as your highest priority.
- Include core conditioning in every workout.
- Remember to engage your core in daily life, especially when lifting.
- Make sure you are turning on your core correctly, gently drawing in your lower abdomen without sucking in around your waist and ribs and breathing normally.
- If you are unsure get some tips from your local physiotherapist.
- Start with simple core exercises and gradually progress them, always making sure quality technique is your priority.
- If you are holding your breath, or adding unwanted moves (such as shrugging your shoulders, tensing your outer abdominals, squeezing your gluteals or clenching your fists) then you are over-challenged.

Perfect posture

As your baby grows, in the second half of your pregnancy your centre of gravity moves forward. Women often compensate by leaning back, leading to the typical sway-back pregnant posture. This is one of the main causes of lower backache in pregnancy. Unfortunately this can create a ricochet effect up your spine, causing a rounded upper back, arched neck and forward-poking chin, all of which are less than optimal and can lead to aches and pains. This is not helped by hormonal changes, joint laxity and the added load on your lower back. It is extremely important that you keep a watch on your posture during this precious time by: keeping your spine long; maintaining your natural lumbar curve (but without leaning back into an exaggerated sway); avoiding shrugging your shoulders; keeping your neck long and in line with your spine; checking you are not locking your knees into a hyper-extended position.

Posture exercise basics:
- During exercise it is important to focus on postural awareness and control.
- Replace sway back with pelvic tilting (see page 77); a fabulous exercise and a healthier way to correct the centre of gravity change rather than leaning back.
- Accommodate for altered balance by avoiding complex choreography, moves or routines.
- Postural awareness and correction, pelvic tilting, back strengthening and core stability exercises all play a role in the prevention and management of back pain.

Keeping cool – monitoring safe and sensible exercise intensity

How hard you should work is a common question, particularly in relation to cardiovascular exercise. It is important to avoid overheating, especially early in your pregnancy and thus you should keep your workout at a low to moderate intensity. Perceived exertion (how you feel when you are exercising) is a great guide to safe intensity: On a scale of 0 to 20, with 1 being at rest and 20 being highly energetic, you should aim to work at a maximal intensity of 12 to 13. Avoid working at a level that has you feeling hot, sweaty or short of breath.

Taking your heart rate is another way to monitor your workout level; traditional guidelines recommend you should not train at heart rates over 140 to 150 beats per minute. Everyone is different so listen to your body and follow the guidelines to ensure the intensity and style of exercises suits you and your situation.

Avoiding overheating exercise basics:
- Keep your perceived exertion at a mild to moderate level. (12 to 13 on a scale of 0 to 20.)
- You should be able to talk during your workout, and you should not feel hot or exhausted.
- 20 to 30 minutes of moderate cardiovascular intensity is plenty. Gentler exercise can be performed for longer.
- Avoid exercising in hot environments, including pools over 28°C.

- Do not exercise if you have a fever.
- Avoid spas and saunas.
- If you have not exercised lately, start gently and build up gradually.
- Sip cool water as you train.
- Take a cool moist face washer with you on warmer days and frequently wipe your wrists and forehead.
- Low-impact exercise is not only better on your joints and pelvic floor, but also less likely to cause you to overheat.

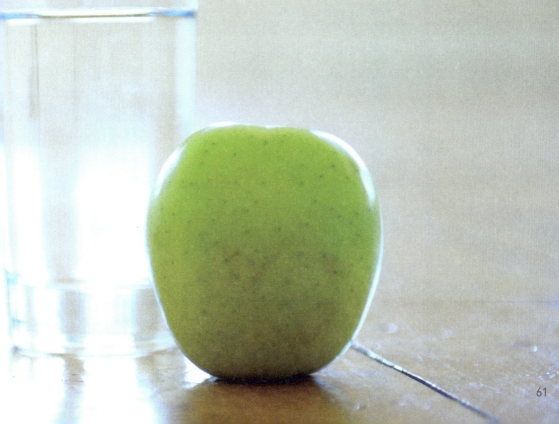

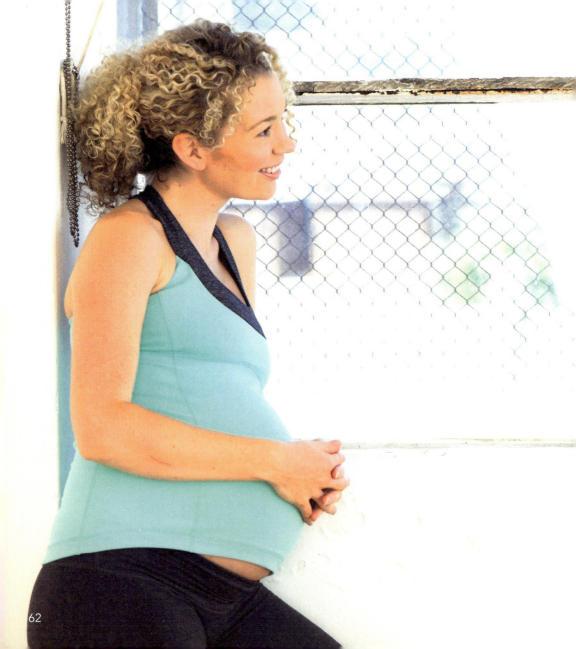

Listening to your body

What type, how hard and how long?

So you are ready to begin your exercise program. Always consult with your healthcare provider before you start to adapt your exercise program to your pregnancy. While you exercise, listen to your body and if something doesn't feel right or is causing discomfort stop the activity and seek advice.

What type?

Low-impact, smooth and controlled exercise styles are ideal. In the interests of looking after your pelvic floor, breast comfort, back and joints avoid high-impact, jolting and straining. Check and correct for great posture and healthy core and pelvic floor recruitment at all times. It is recommended you avoid contact sports and activities that involve a high risk of falls or blows to the abdomen. You will benefit from including a range of exercise styles into your repertoire, such as low-impact cardiovascular exercise, low-load strength training mobility, flexibility and relaxation, plus your all-important posture, core and pelvic exercises.

How hard?

There are several reasons why mums-to-be are encouraged to exercise at a mild to moderate level. This is less stressful on both your body and your baby. It avoids overheating due to raised core temperature, joint and pelvic floor stress. How much you can do within this moderate intensity depends on your fitness, but as a guide, on an exercise intensity scale of 0 to 20, you should feel like you are working at around 12 to 13.

How long?

The duration of your training needs to be balanced with the intensity. If you are taking a leisurely walk, you may be quite comfortable to go for an hour, whereas 20 minutes will be plenty when working more intensely; on a stationary bike, for example. Everyone is different; if you are used to exercise you will probably be quite comfortable with a moderate cardiovascular session of 20 to 30 minutes, followed by low-load strength conditioning for another 20 minutes, but if you are commencing a fitness plan you should start with 5 to 10 minutes and build up slowly. As a guide, when you finish you should feel like you have exercised but not be absolutely worn out. Everyone is different so listen to your body and follow the guidelines to ensure the intensity and style of exercises suits you and your situation.

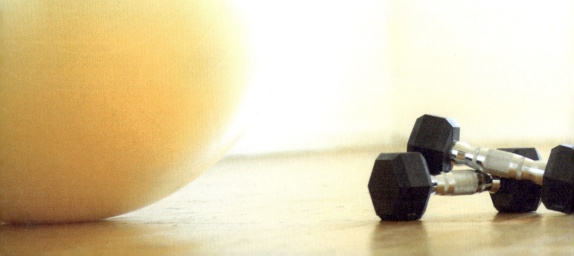

Training tips

Following are general guidelines to help you towards developing a safe and effective pregnancy fitness program.

- Start lightly and progress gradually if you have been previously sedentary or you have had several weeks of rest.
- Exercise regularly, about 3 to 5 times per week.
- Include a mix of moderate low-impact cardiovascular exercise, strength training, pregnancy-specific exercise, mobility, flexibility and relaxation.
- Monitor the intensity of your workout as above.
- Sip water before, during and after exercise.
- Ensure smooth, controlled technique when exercising, avoiding any bouncing, jolting or an extreme range of movement.
- Avoid contact sport during your pregnancy.
- Vary your exercise routine to keep things interesting.
- Include pelvic floor, core stability and postural training.
- Prioritise posture and core stability during strength exercise and check that your weights are at a level that allows you to breathe with ease.
- It is important to include stretching at the end of a workout to maintain muscle length and flexibility.
- Stretch within comfort and normal range of movement.
- Complement your pregnancy fitness program with a healthy, fresh diet, lots of water and plenty of sleep.
- Include relaxation (see page 195–198) – half an hour while resting or going to sleep, or five minutes after your exercise session. These techniques will come in handy during labour and the early weeks of motherhood.

If in doubt, leave it out. Avoid exercises that you are unsure about for the safety of you and your baby.

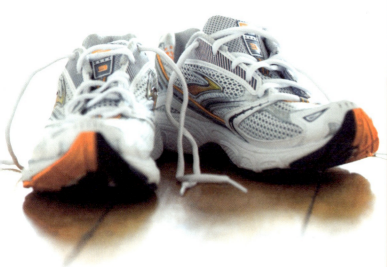
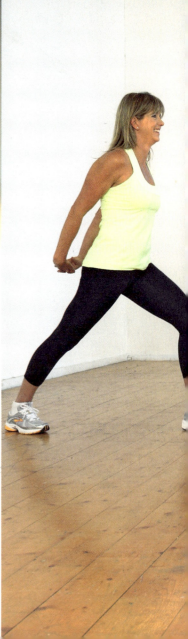

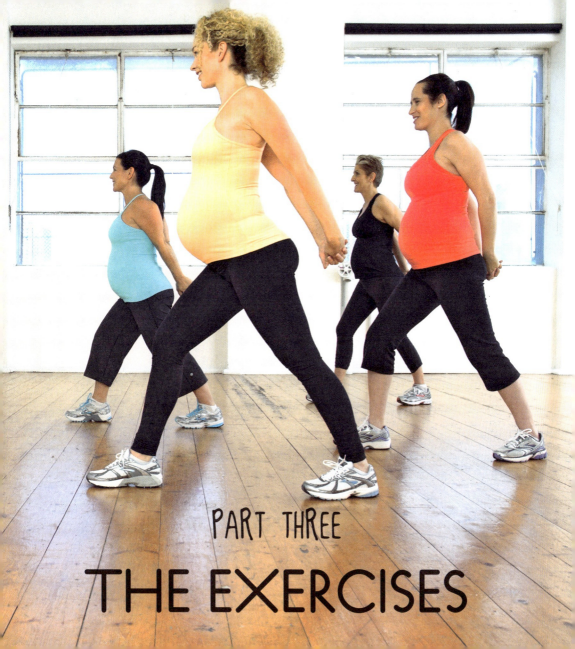

Safe and effective exercise to suit your goals and pregnancy

The following exercises are designed to suit different fitness levels and stages of pregnancy. Exercise styles to help you maintain general fitness include mobility, cardiovascular fitness, strength and flexibility. In addition you will find a selection of important pregnancy specific exercises such as pelvic floor and core training, postural exercises, labour preparation and relaxation techniques as well as tips for when you go to the gym, exercise in the water or attend group exercise classes. Choose from the range of options to design your own training plan or refer to the exercise programs at the end of the book to select a program that suits your situation and goals. Equipment such as fitballs, hand weights and resistance bands, that can be used at home, are included in some exercises but there are plenty of non-equipment choices also. Next to the exercises you will see 'technique tips', 'modifications' and 'progressions', allowing you to fine-tune your form as well as lighten or raise the challenge to suit your fitness and ability. For those with pregnancy-related concerns check the 'extra care' point for modifications to suit your needs.

> Always check with your doctor before commencing an exercise program and seek professional advice if you experience any discomfort or concern.

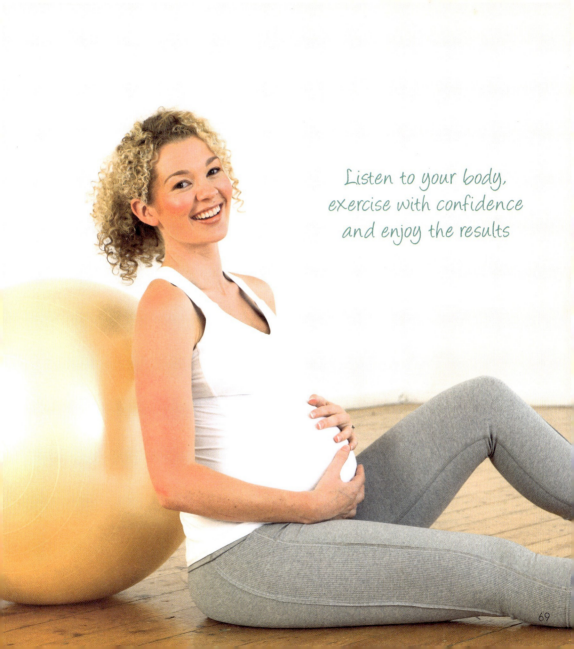

Listen to your body, exercise with confidence and enjoy the results

Mobility exercises

Gentle rhythmical movements help minimise joint stiffness and maintain full range of movement. Mobility exercises are fabulous during pregnancy to help prevent or manage backache, aid blood-flow, and are an important inclusion to your exercise program. For women who have been advised to rest during their pregnancy they serve as a gentle exercise option to assist circulation and the maintenance of muscle tone as well as avoid stiffness that can be associated with inactivity. For those of you who are more active, mobility exercises will be an integral part of your warm-up or cool down and you will find they also help relieve feelings of tiredness or stiffness throughout your day.

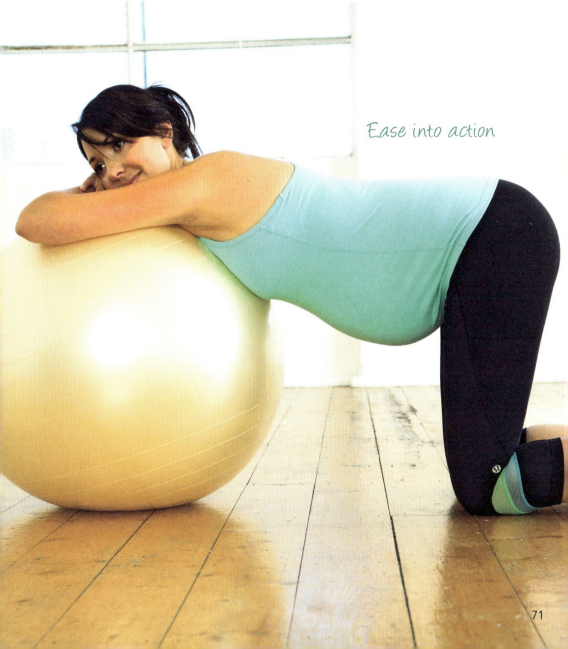

Ease into action

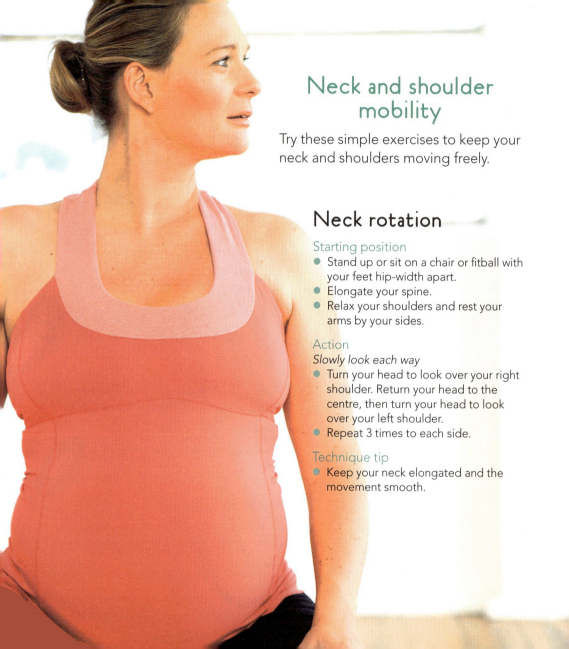

Neck and shoulder mobility

Try these simple exercises to keep your neck and shoulders moving freely.

Neck rotation

Starting position
- Stand up or sit on a chair or fitball with your feet hip-width apart.
- Elongate your spine.
- Relax your shoulders and rest your arms by your sides.

Action
Slowly look each way
- Turn your head to look over your right shoulder. Return your head to the centre, then turn your head to look over your left shoulder.
- Repeat 3 times to each side.

Technique tip
- Keep your neck elongated and the movement smooth.

Neck semi-circle

Starting position
- Stand up or sit on a chair or fitball with your feet hip-width apart.
- Elongate your spine.
- Relax your shoulders and rest your arms by your sides.

Action
Draw a semi-circle with your chin
- Turn your head to look over your right shoulder, then slowly tilt your head to look down at your right hip, taking your chin to your chest.
- Make a slow semi-circle, bringing your chin across your chest until it reaches your left shoulder. Lengthen your neck until you are looking over your left shoulder.
- Reverse the movement.
- Repeat 3 times each way.

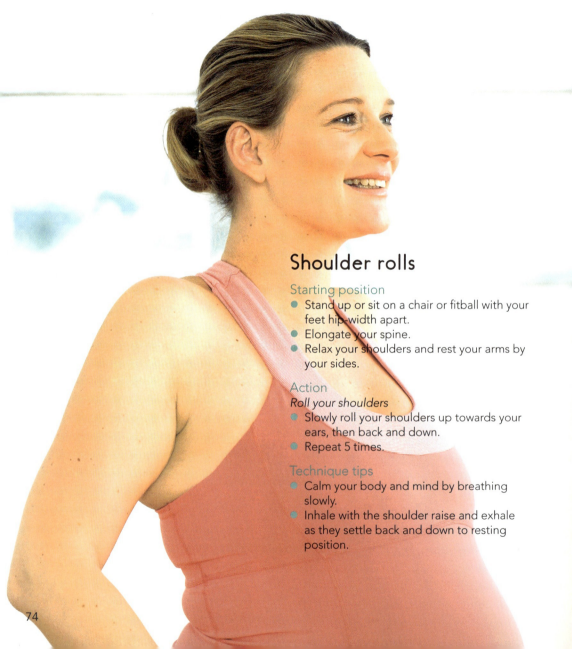

Shoulder rolls

Starting position
- Stand up or sit on a chair or fitball with your feet hip-width apart.
- Elongate your spine.
- Relax your shoulders and rest your arms by your sides.

Action
Roll your shoulders
- Slowly roll your shoulders up towards your ears, then back and down.
- Repeat 5 times.

Technique tips
- Calm your body and mind by breathing slowly.
- Inhale with the shoulder raise and exhale as they settle back and down to resting position.

Swim to the sky

Starting position
- Stand up or sit on a chair or fitball with your feet hip-width apart.
- Elongate your spine.
- Relax your shoulders and rest your arms by your sides.

Action
Reach up and out
- Inhale as you bring your hands side by side. Move them up in front of the midline of your body, palms passing close to your face.
- Reach to the sky, then turn your palms outwards.
- Exhale as you separate your palms, reaching your arms out and down sideways, creating a large circle to end with your arms down by your side.
- Repeat 5 times.

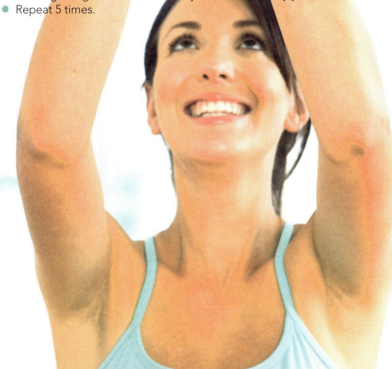

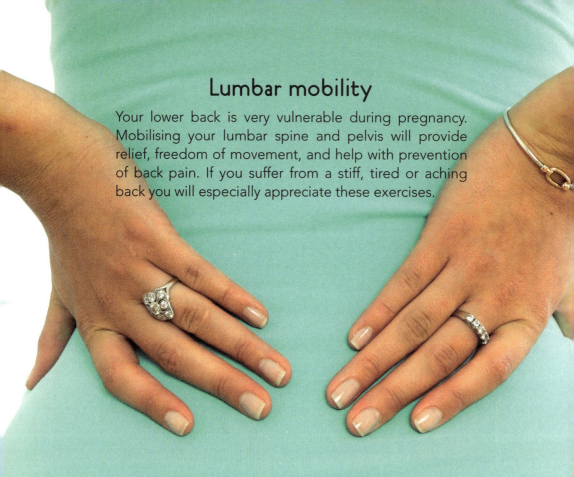

Lumbar mobility

Your lower back is very vulnerable during pregnancy. Mobilising your lumbar spine and pelvis will provide relief, freedom of movement, and help with prevention of back pain. If you suffer from a stiff, tired or aching back you will especially appreciate these exercises.

Ease away the tension in your lower back

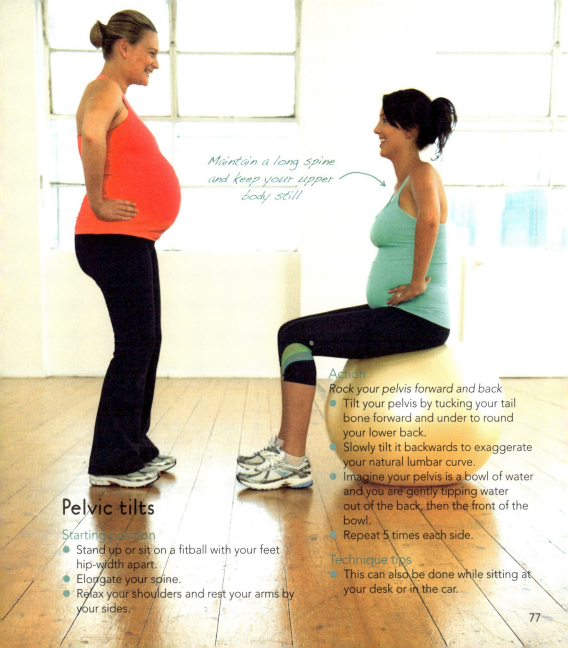

Maintain a long spine and keep your upper body still

Pelvic tilts

Starting position
- Stand up or sit on a fitball with your feet hip-width apart.
- Elongate your spine.
- Relax your shoulders and rest your arms by your sides.

Action:
Rock your pelvis forward and back
- Tilt your pelvis by tucking your tail bone forward and under to round your lower back.
- Slowly tilt it backwards to exaggerate your natural lumbar curve.
- Imagine your pelvis is a bowl of water and you are gently tipping water out of the back, then the front of the bowl.
- Repeat 5 times each side.

Technique tips
- This can also be done while sitting at your desk or in the car.

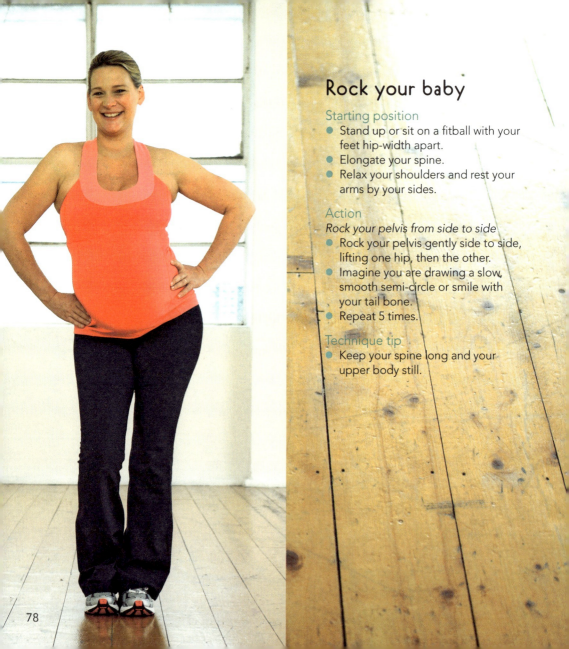

Rock your baby

Starting position
- Stand up or sit on a fitball with your feet hip-width apart.
- Elongate your spine.
- Relax your shoulders and rest your arms by your sides.

Action
Rock your pelvis from side to side
- Rock your pelvis gently side to side, lifting one hip, then the other.
- Imagine you are drawing a slow, smooth semi-circle or smile with your tail bone.
- Repeat 5 times.

Technique tip
- Keep your spine long and your upper body still.

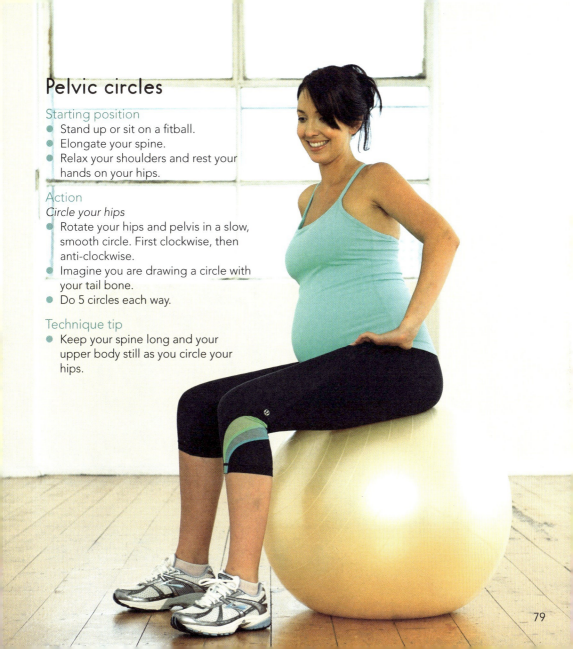

Pelvic circles

Starting position
- Stand up or sit on a fitball.
- Elongate your spine.
- Relax your shoulders and rest your hands on your hips.

Action
Circle your hips
- Rotate your hips and pelvis in a slow, smooth circle. First clockwise, then anti-clockwise.
- Imagine you are drawing a circle with your tail bone.
- Do 5 circles each way.

Technique tip
- Keep your spine long and your upper body still as you circle your hips.

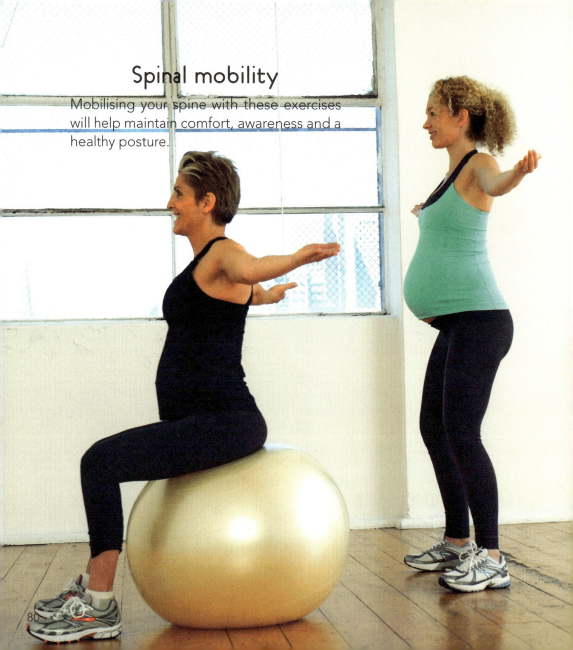

Spinal mobility

Mobilising your spine with these exercises will help maintain comfort, awareness and a healthy posture.

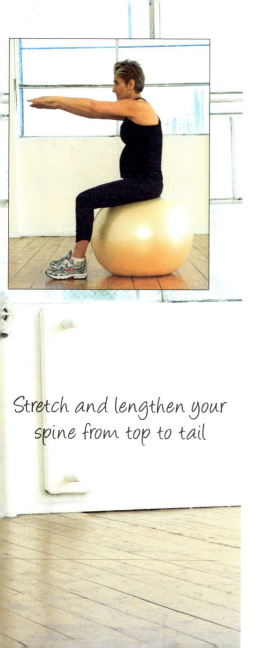

Stretch and lengthen your spine from top to tail

Round and open

Starting position
- Stand up or sit on a fitball with your feet hip-width apart.
- Elongate your spine.
- Relax your shoulders and rest your arms by your sides.

Action
Round and straighten your back
- Inhale and raise your arms sideways to shoulder height.
- Exhale and bring your hands forward, thumbs down, to meet in front of your chest.
- Feel your shoulder blades glide forward on your ribs as you round your upper back.
- At the same time, tuck your tail bone in and under, rounding your lower back.
- Imagine you are creating a 'c' curve with your whole spine.
- Turn your palms upwards and inhale as you open your arms wide again, lengthening your neck and spine back to return to upright position.
- Repeat 5 times.

Technique tip
- Your sternum (chest bone) moves backward as you round your spine and forward as you open your arms and lengthen your spine.

Roll and reach

Starting position
- Sit on a fitball.
- Elongate your spine.
- Relax your shoulders and rest your arms by your sides.

Action
Round your back, swim to the sky, lean forward and roll back up
- Inhale and raise your arms sideways to shoulder height.
- Exhale and bring your hands forward, thumbs down, to meet in front of your chest.
- Feel your shoulder blades glide forward on your ribs as you round your upper back, rolling the fitball slightly forward. Become as round as you can, as though you are hugging a ball.
- Return to upright sitting, bringing your hands into your chest.
- Inhale and reach for the sky. Imagine yourself long and tall as you reach upwards.
- Exhale as you hinge forward from the hips, rolling the ball backwards. Keep your back straight and rest your hands on your thighs.
- Inhale as you slowly round your spine and roll back to upright posture.
- Repeat 3 times.

Technique tips
- Roll up vertebra by vertebra, starting at your tail bone and finishing sitting upright.

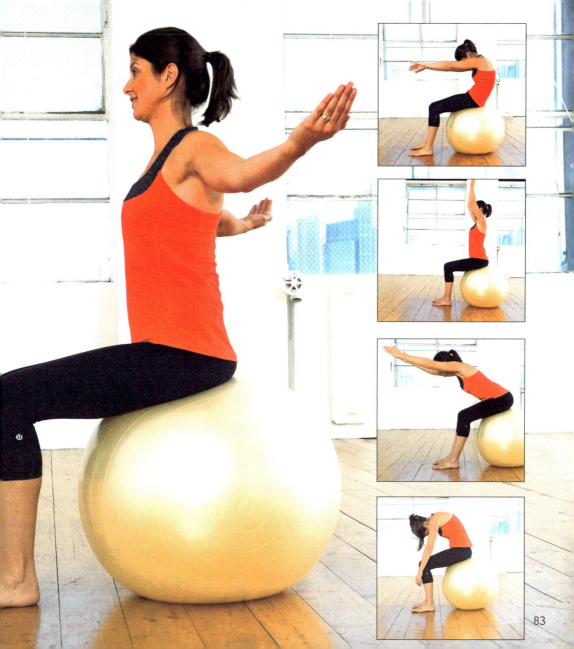

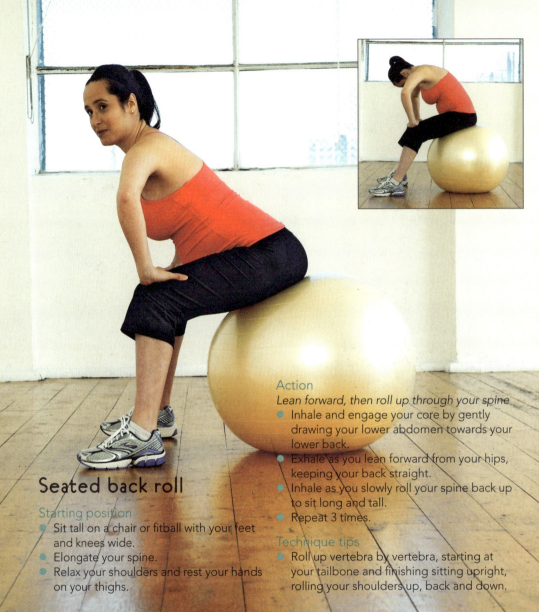

Seated back roll

Starting position
- Sit tall on a chair or fitball with your feet and knees wide.
- Elongate your spine.
- Relax your shoulders and rest your hands on your thighs.

Action
Lean forward, then roll up through your spine
- Inhale and engage your core by gently drawing your lower abdomen towards your lower back.
- Exhale as you lean forward from your hips, keeping your back straight.
- Inhale as you slowly roll your spine back up to sit long and tall.
- Repeat 3 times.

Technique tips
- Roll up vertebra by vertebra, starting at your tailbone and finishing sitting upright, rolling your shoulders up, back and down.

Cat curl

Starting position
- Kneeling on all fours with your back straight.
- Keep your back straight without arching it.

Action
Round your back
- Slowly round your back upwards then lower back down to the starting position.
- Repeat 5 times.

Technique tip
- Avoid arching your back.

Extra care
- If you do not like to kneel on all fours due to reflux, perform 'Round and Open' exercise page 81.
- If you have wrist discomfort, rest your upper arms across a fitball instead.

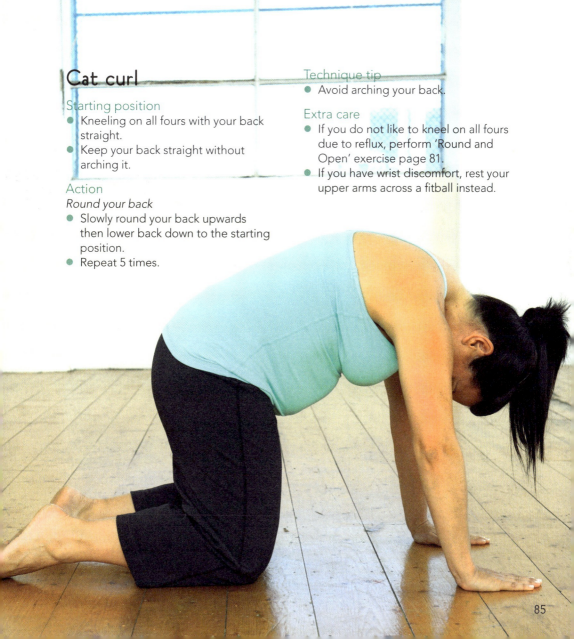

Disco cat

Starting position
- Kneeling on all fours.

Action
Circle your back
- Move your torso in a slow circular motion around its axis.
- Gently lower your tummy towards the floor, then take your body to one side, then to round back and finally the other side.
- Repeat 5 circles in each direction.

Extra care
- If you do not like to kneel on all fours due to reflux or wrist discomfort, try 'Pelvic Circles' exercise page 79.
- Leaning on a fitball or sitting up is preferable if you have wrist discomfort.

Your midsection moves up, sideways, down and around.

Foot and ankle mobility

Putting your feet up and performing mobilising exercise takes the load of your legs, back and pelvic floor and helps to relieve stiffness and swelling. These exercises are particularly helpful in maintaining mobility and muscle function when you are unable to do more active exercise.

Ankle circles

Starting position
- Sitting with your feet up on a foot stool, couch or bed.

Action
Circle your feet
- Move both feet clockwise, drawing large circles with your toes but keep your legs still. Repeat in an anti-clockwise direction.
- Repeat 5 to 10 times clockwise and anti-clockwise.

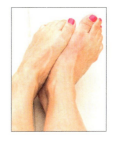

Calf pumps

Starting position
- Sitting with your feet up on a foot stool, couch or bed.

Action
Wave your feet
- Point and flex your feet as though waving them up and down.
- Repeat 10 times.

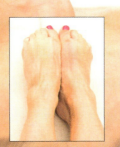 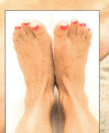

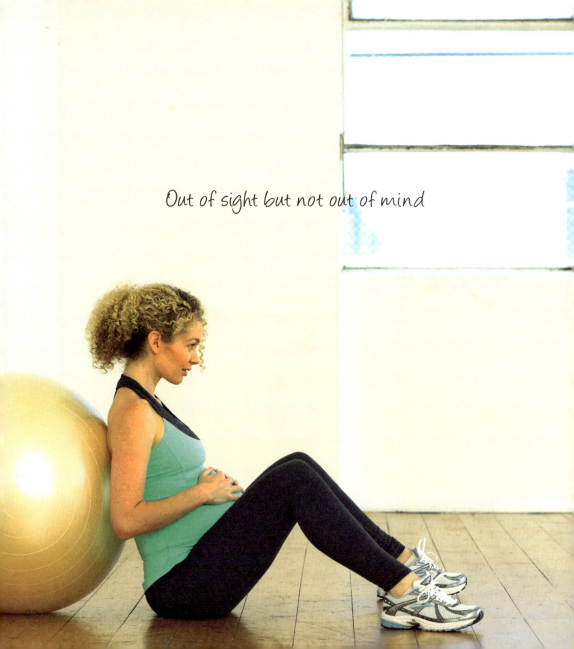

Pelvic floor training

Sound pelvic floor exercise technique involves lifting the muscles as though lifting your baby towards your heart, while keeping other muscles relaxed. You should be aware of an internal sensation of the pelvic floor muscles lifting without seeing or feeling outer muscle activity. It will feel similar to when you are trying to avoid passing wind or hold on when you need to go to the toilet.

Unfortunately many women unknowingly 'push down' when they should be lifting their pelvic floor. This is detrimental to its strength, so make sure you feel an upwards, lifting sensation rather than a bearing down or pushing sensation. Squeezing gluteal (bottom) muscles, and breath holding are two common yet incorrect techniques. Keep all your other muscles relaxed; shoulder shrugging, bracing your abdominals, making fists and curling your toes will not help your pelvic floor get stronger! While you will find sitting and standing convenient positions for exercising your pelvic floor, you need these muscles to be strong all day, every day so practise pelvic-floor exercises in a range of positions.

Take time to follow the pelvic-floor instructions carefully and if you are in doubt about your technique or have concern, a visit to a women's health and continence physiotherapist will be invaluable.

Technique matters

Don't add stress to an already compromised muscle group

The vital rule of good prenatal fitness is to avoid exercises and activities that stress your pelvic floor. High impact activities such as running and jumping are detrimental due to the bouncing action of your baby and uterus. Anything that causes strain via increased pressure will have a weakening effect on your pelvic floor muscles. Heavy lifting or pushing, especially if you hold your breath, should be avoided. It is important to avoid straining your muscles when you go to the toilet, especially if you are suffering constipation. Take your time, enjoy a healthy, high-fibre diet and drink plenty of water.

Don't harm your pelvic floor with:

- high impact exercise
- bouncy jolty activities
- high load, heavy lifting
- standing for prolonged periods of time, especially late in pregnancy
- activities that have you holding your breath and 'straining'.

Don't stress your pelvic floor with these exercises:

- running, jumping, star jumps
- abdominal curls and sit-ups
- lifting heavy weights
- hovers / planks
- double leg raises
- wide squats and lunges.

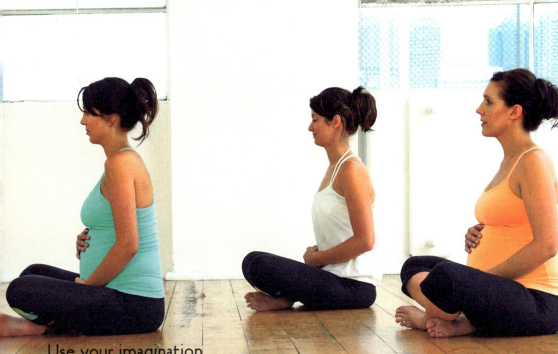

Use your imagination

Different cues and images work for different people when learning correct pelvic floor technique, including:
- Imagine you are stopping the flow of urine while going to the toilet.
- Imagine you are trying to avoid passing wind. Draw inwards around your back passage, then bring that 'muscle lift' through from your tail bone forward to your pubic bone as though you are also needing to control your bladder.
- Imagine lifting your baby towards your heart with your pelvic floor.
- Imagine you are trying to squeeze your partner during sex.
- Visualise the space within your pelvis. Use your deep muscles as though trying to make this space smaller.

Pelvic-floor exercise basics

Mix and match the following exercises for a varied and functional pelvic floor fitness program.

Comfortable starting positions

The following are all great options for training your pelvic floor. You can pretty much practise your pelvic-floor training anywhere at any time.

- Sitting tall on a chair or fitball, arms relaxed by your sides or hands resting on your thighs, or leaning forward with your arms resting on your thighs.
- Sitting cross-legged on the floor.
- Standing tall.
- Kneeling upright or sitting back on your heels.
- Kneeling and resting your chest and arms on a fitball.
- Lying on your side.
- While you are walking.

When doing your pelvic-floor exercises, always elongate your spine and maintain the natural curve of your lower back. Don't tense up, keep every part of your body relaxed – except for your pelvic-floor – and remember to breathe normally.

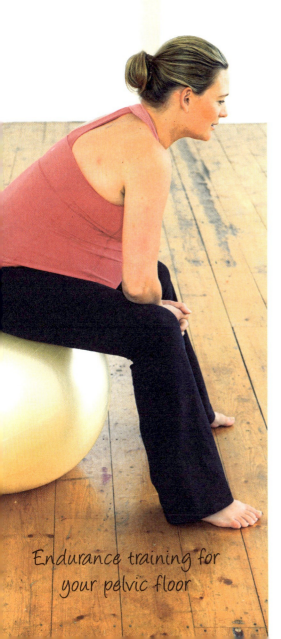

Endurance training for your pelvic floor

Pelvic-floor long hold

Starting position
- Choose from the list on page 92.

Action
Lift and hold
- Imagine the muscular floor of your pelvis running from your tail bone to your pubic bone.
- Lift your pelvic floor at the back as if you are trying to avoid passing wind, and then continue the lift forward to your pubic bone as if you also need to control your bladder.
- Hold this maximal pelvic-floor lift for 5 breaths and then rest for 5 breaths.
- Repeat 3 times.
- Gradually increase the time to holding for 10 breaths and relaxing for 10 breaths as your control and strength improve. Ideally you will eventually be able to hold your pelvic floor contraction for 60 seconds, although this may be difficult during pregnancy.

Technique tips
- Aim for maximal pelvic floor contraction, lifting it as high as you can while maintaining normal breathing.
- Relax any other unwanted muscle tension, for example your buttocks.

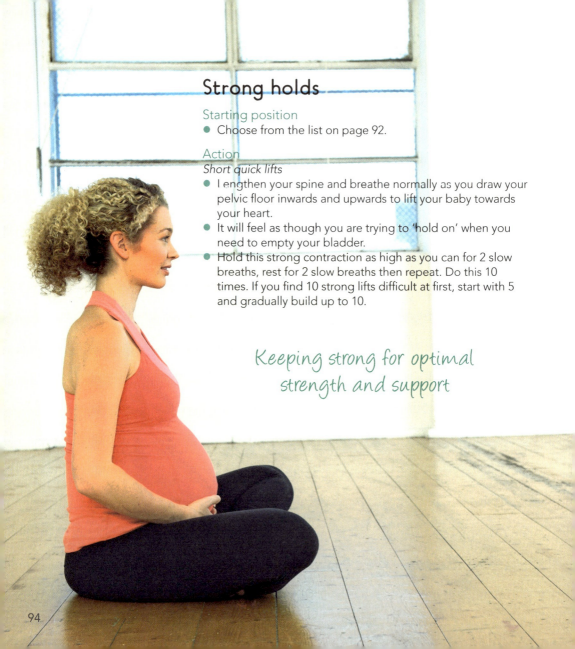

Strong holds

Starting position
- Choose from the list on page 92.

Action
Short quick lifts
- Lengthen your spine and breathe normally as you draw your pelvic floor inwards and upwards to lift your baby towards your heart.
- It will feel as though you are trying to 'hold on' when you need to empty your bladder.
- Hold this strong contraction as high as you can for 2 slow breaths, rest for 2 slow breaths then repeat. Do this 10 times. If you find 10 strong lifts difficult at first, start with 5 and gradually build up to 10.

Keeping strong for optimal strength and support

Quick lifts

Starting position
- Choose from the list on page 92.

Action
Short quick lifts
- Be aware of your pelvic floor working like a strong hammock within your pelvis.
- Lift it quickly and with maximal strength for 2 seconds then release the hold for the same amount of time.
- Continue to raise and release, performing continual strong quick lifting and lowering of your pelvic floor. Repeat 10 times or more if you can.

For confidence when you sneeze, cough, jump and laugh

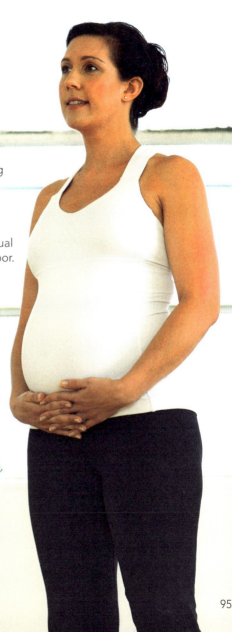

Strong hold plus quick lifts

Performing a maximal pelvic floor lift and then superimposing three quick lifts is a more challenging, but very effective technique. Try this if you have managed the previous three exercise styles easily.

Starting position
- Choose from the list on page 92.

Action
A strong lift with quick lifts on top
- Lengthen your spine and breathe normally as you draw your pelvic floor inwards and upwards to lift your baby towards your heart.
- Hold a maximum lift, then add 3 quick strong lifts.
- Relax your pelvic floor. Repeat the whole exercise 5 times.

Combining techniques for excellent control

Relax your pelvic floor

Starting position
- Choose from the list on page 92.

Action
Lift your pelvic floor then consciously let it relax
- Lengthen your spine and breathe normally as you draw your pelvic floor inwards and upwards to lift your baby towards your heart.
- Hold for 3 to 5 slow breaths.
- Now slowly and consciously lower your pelvic floor, feeling it relax back to its resting position. Try not to 'push' it down.
- Relax for 3 to 5 breaths. Repeat 10 times.

Training tips
- Become aware of how it feels to consciously relax your pelvic floor.
- Replace this as one of your 3 pelvic floor sessions during the third trimester.

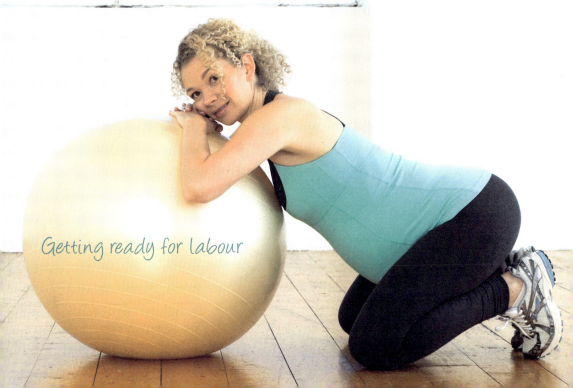

Getting ready for labour

Posture

Keep your body happy and healthy by checking and correcting your posture throughout the day.

Keep an eye on your posture when you are exercising. Make sure you maintain good alignment of the body parts that are still, as well as maintaining a smooth technique for those that are moving. Avoid bad habits such as sway or rounded low back, slouched or shrugged shoulders and hyperextended knees. Instead, maintain natural spinal curves, long neck, shoulders relaxed back and down and soft knees.

Posture perfect for a healthy pregnancy

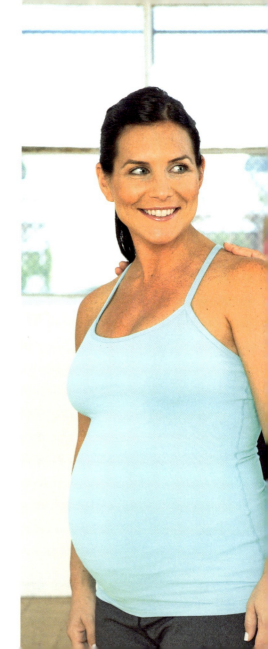

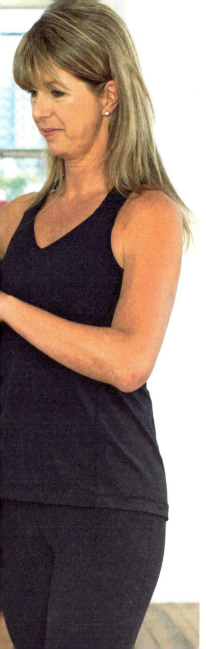

Gold and silver threads

Starting position
- Stand tall with your feet hip-width apart.
- Elongate your spine.
- Relax your shoulders, rest your arms by your sides.

Action
Lengthen your spine, relax your shoulders
- Spread your weight evenly across your feet and toes.
- Soften your knees.
- Lightly draw your lower abdomen towards your lower back to engage your core muscles and lift your pelvic floor.
- Breathe naturally as you imagine a golden thread running from your tail bone, through every vertebra and out the top of your head, elongating your spine upwards.
- Now imagine two silver threads running from the base of your shoulder blades, gently pulling downwards and inwards to your tail bone.
- Hold for 3 slow breaths.
- Perform this quick posture check before and during exercises and whenever you think of it during the day.

Technique tips
- Breathe normally.
- Check the natural curve of your lower back is present but not exaggerated.
- Check your shoulders remain relaxed.
- Your head should feel light and your neck long.
- Think of lengthening your waist.
- Imagine you are increasing the distance between each vertebra.

core strength and stability

Strong core muscles are like the foundations of your house. Although out of sight, they are a vital element for support and maintenance of healthy function. During pregnancy core stability is important for back health, as well as supporting your baby and your pelvis. Core strength replaces outer abdominal work during pregnancy and deserves high priority. You should always engage your core whenever you do any exercise, before lifting and whenever you think of it during the day. Don't rush into core strengthening – progress through the following stages. Once you have established good core muscle technique you can then add movement or a fitball to further challenge stability and control.

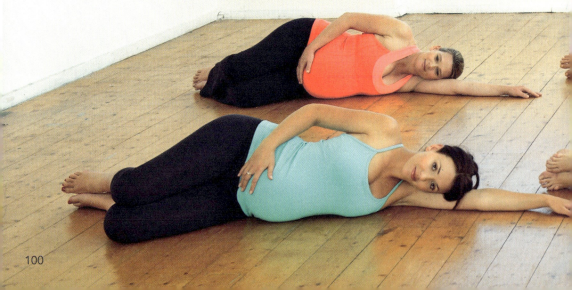

Core control in side-lying

Starting position
- Lie on your side with your legs bent and your head, neck and shoulders relaxed.
- Rest your top hand on your lower abdomen.
- Breathe normally.

Action
Engage your deep abdominals
- Gently draw your lower abdomen towards your lower back as though hugging your baby with your deep abdominals. Hold this for 3 to 5 slow breaths.
- Repeat 5 times.

Progressions
- Progress from lying, to kneeling, to sitting then standing developing good technique in each position.

Extra care
- If you suffer from reflux you will prefer the seated or standing positions rather than lying down.
- If you have pelvic-joint pain, take care getting up and down off the floor, keep your feet and knees together as though you are wearing a miniskirt.

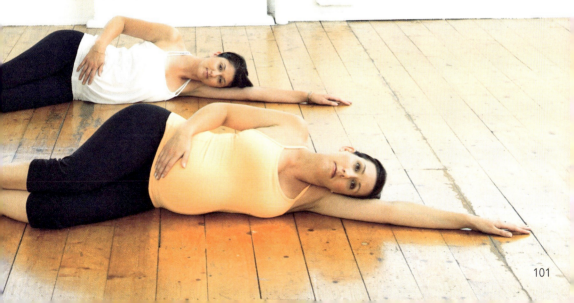

Core control with four-point kneeling

Starting position
- Kneeling on all fours, with your hands under shoulders and knees under hips.
- Soften your elbows, drawing your shoulders towards your tail bone.
- Elongate your spine and keep your back straight while still maintaining the natural curve in your back. Look down at the floor to keep your neck in line with your spine.

Action
Draw your bikini area towards your lower back
- Breathing normally, gently draw your lower abdomen away from the floor, lifting your baby towards your back. Imagine you are drawing your bikini line towards your lower back.
- Hold for 5 breaths and relax.
- Repeat 5 times.

Training tips
- Avoid dropping into sway back or rounding your upper back

Progressions
- Four-point kneeling with single arm and or leg raises will further challenge your core control and add extra back strengthening. See page 104.

Extra care
- If you have carpal tunnel syndrome or leaning through your wrists causes discomfort you can do this resting your arms and upper body on a fitball.
- If you do not like to be horizontal due to gastric reflux you may prefer the upright core options.
- If you have pelvic-joint pain, take care getting up and down off the floor, keep your feet and knees together as though you are wearing a miniskirt.

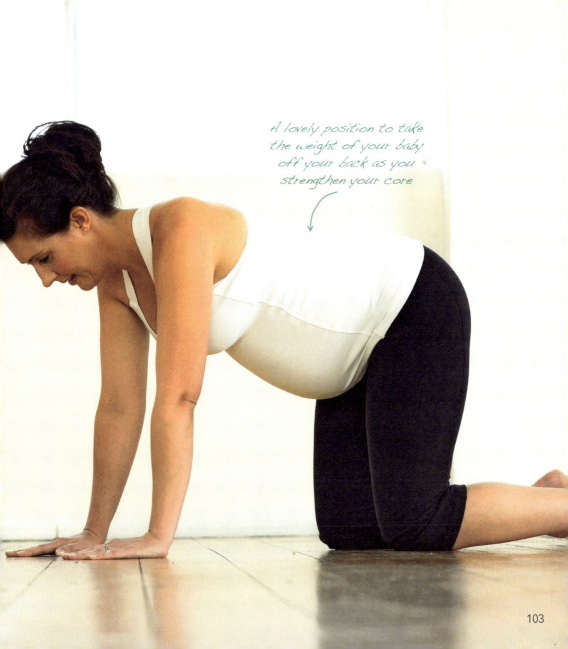

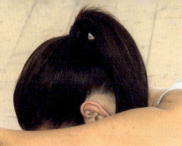

Four-point kneeling with arm or leg raise

Starting position
- Kneeling on all fours, with your hands under shoulders and knees under hips.
- Soften your elbows, drawing your shoulders towards your tail bone.
- Elongate your spine and keep your back straight while still maintaining the natural curve in your back. Look down at the floor to keep your neck in line with your spine.

Action
Raise your arm forward
- Breathing normally, gently draw your lower abdomen away from the floor, lifting your baby towards your back.
- Reach your arm up and forward until it is level with your shoulder beside your ear.
- Hold for 3 to 5 breaths then relax and repeat raising your left arm.
- Repeat 5 times on each arm.

Technique tips
- Keep your back straight and stable by maintaining the natural curve in your spine.
- Keep your neck in line with your spine.
- Avoid shrugging your shoulder as you raise your arm.

Modifications
- Slowly alternate lifting one hand then the other just off the floor.

Extra care
- If leaning through your wrist is uncomfortable opt for seated core or fitball wall hover instead (pages 106 and 115).
- If you do not like to be horizontal due to gastric reflux you may prefer the fitball wall hover on page 115.

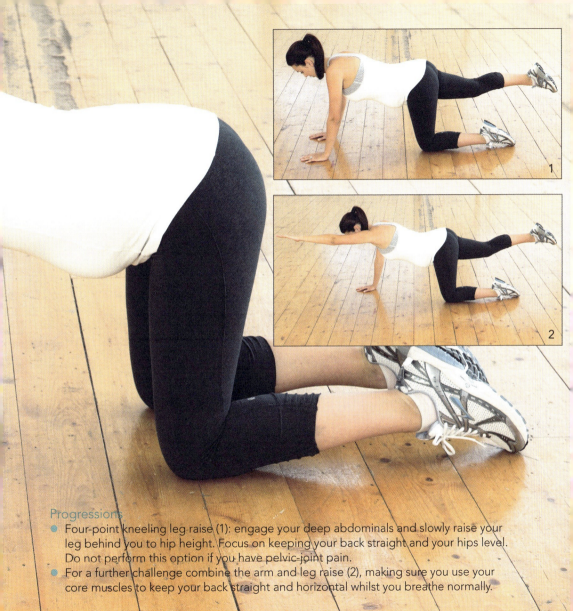

Progressions
- Four-point kneeling leg raise (1): engage your deep abdominals and slowly raise your leg behind you to hip height. Focus on keeping your back straight and your hips level. Do not perform this option if you have pelvic-joint pain.
- For a further challenge combine the arm and leg raise (2), making sure you use your core muscles to keep your back straight and horizontal whilst you breathe normally.

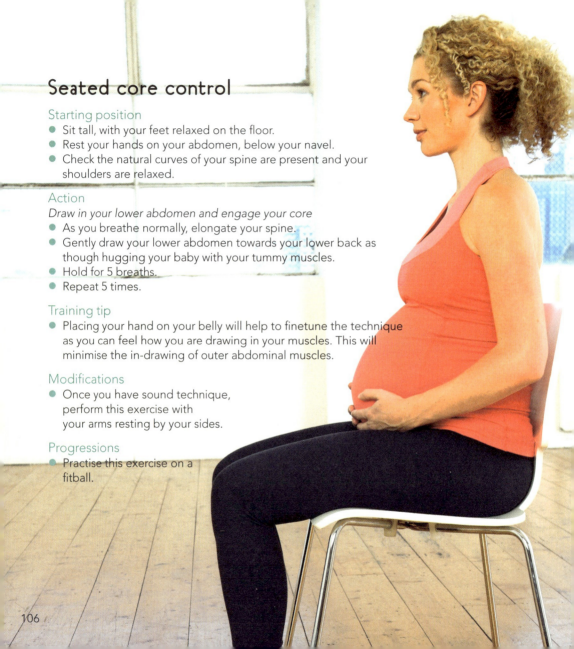

Seated core control

Starting position
- Sit tall, with your feet relaxed on the floor.
- Rest your hands on your abdomen, below your navel.
- Check the natural curves of your spine are present and your shoulders are relaxed.

Action
Draw in your lower abdomen and engage your core
- As you breathe normally, elongate your spine.
- Gently draw your lower abdomen towards your lower back as though hugging your baby with your tummy muscles.
- Hold for 5 breaths.
- Repeat 5 times.

Training tip
- Placing your hand on your belly will help to finetune the technique as you can feel how you are drawing in your muscles. This will minimise the in-drawing of outer abdominal muscles.

Modifications
- Once you have sound technique, perform this exercise with your arms resting by your sides.

Progressions
- Practise this exercise on a fitball.

Standing core control

Starting position
- Stand tall with your feet hip-width apart.
- Relax your shoulders and rest your arms by your sides.

Action
Draw in below your navel
- As you breathe normally, elongate your spine.
- Gently draw your lower abdomen towards your lower back as though hugging your baby with your tummy muscles.
- Hold for 5 breaths.
- Repeat 5 times.

Technique tips
- Do not be surprised if you feel your pelvic floor lift. This indicates you have good technique and awareness because the muscles work together.
- Avoid the temptation of sucking in your ribs and tummy as this switches on outer abdominals and makes it harder for the deep ones to work. You should not see rib or chest movement.

Wall lean and reach

Starting position
- Stand with your feet about 1 metre away for the wall.
- Place your hands on the wall as you incline forward keeping your hips and back straight.
- Check that your hands are level with your shoulders. Your fingers pointing upwards and your elbows are slightly bent.

Action
Leaning on the wall raise one arm then the other.
- Elongate your spine and relax your shoulders.
- Draw your shoulder blades down and your lower abdomen inwards as though hugging your baby with your deep abdominals.
- Slowly slide one hand up and off the wall to raise your arm by your ear.
- Hold for 3 to 5 breaths.
- Repeat 3 times on each arm.

Technique tips
- Keep your back and hips straight.
- Do not bend at the hips, arch your back or shrug your shoulders.
- As you raise your arm ensure your shoulder blade stays down.

Extra care
- If you have carpal tunnel syndrome or do not like leaning through your wrists replace with the fitball wall hover on page 115.

Modifications
- Initially you may like to hold the position, keeping both hands on the wall for 3 slow breaths, walk in to relax and then repeat 5 times.
- Gradually progress to simply sliding your hand slowly up and down without taking it off the wall.

Progressions
- Add a leg raise, lifting your opposite foot just a little off the floor to extend your leg behind you. This exercise is not appropriate if you have pelvic joint pain.
- The wall push-up (pages 164–165) is another progression for this exercise.

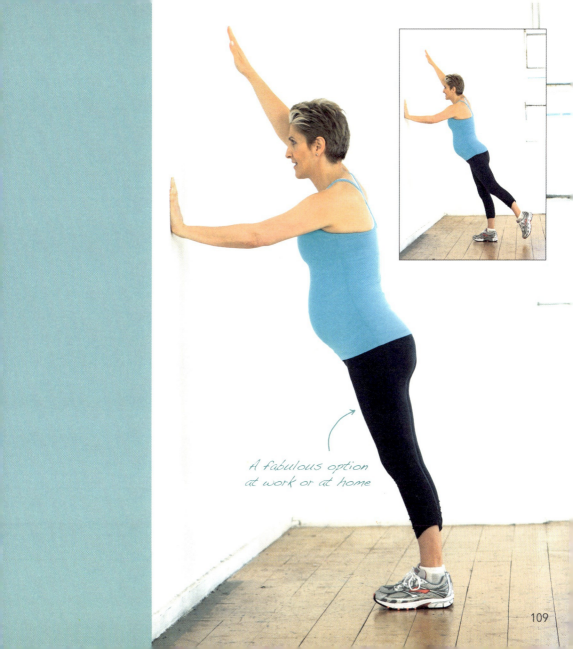

A fabulous option at work or at home

Supine leg slide

This core control exercise is appropriate during the first 16 weeks only.

Starting position
- Lying on your back with your hands resting on your hips.
- Bend your knees so that your heels are aligned with your sit bones.
- Notice the position of your lower back on the floor. Your goal is to maintain this position when you move your leg.

Action
Keep your back straight as you slide your heel away
- Elongate your spine on the floor, breathe normally and relax your neck, shoulders and arms.
- Engage your core, gently drawing your lower abdomen towards the floor.
- Now slowly slide one heel along the floor, until your leg is resting straight. Return your leg back to the bent knee position and repeat on the other side.
- Repeat 5 times on each leg.

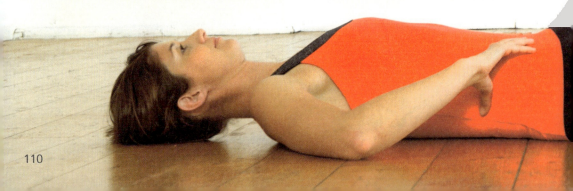

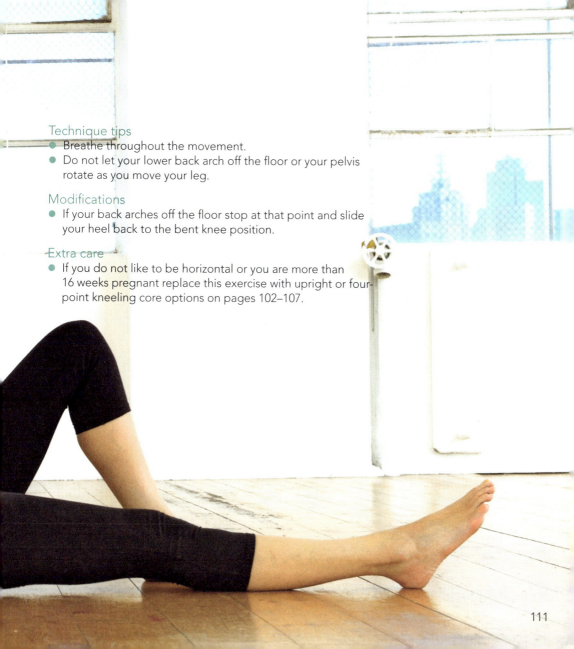

Technique tips
- Breathe throughout the movement.
- Do not let your lower back arch off the floor or your pelvis rotate as you move your leg.

Modifications
- If your back arches off the floor stop at that point and slide your heel back to the bent knee position.

Extra care
- If you do not like to be horizontal or you are more than 16 weeks pregnant replace this exercise with upright or four-point kneeling core options on pages 102–107.

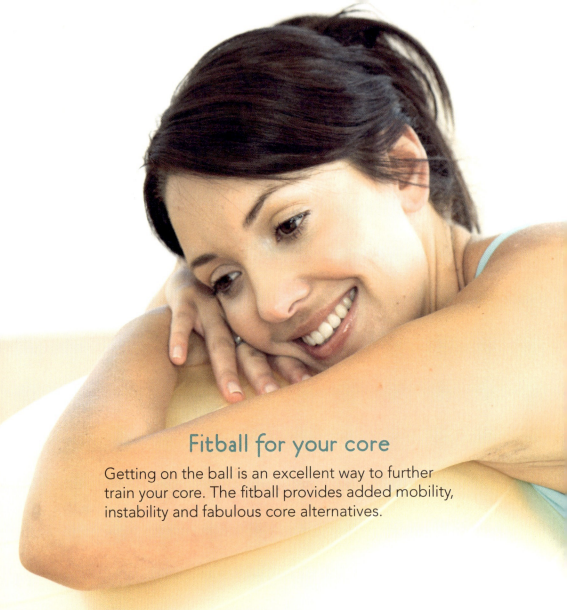

Fitball for your core

Getting on the ball is an excellent way to further train your core. The fitball provides added mobility, instability and fabulous core alternatives.

Seated leg raise

Starting position
- Sit tall on a fitball, with your feet hip-width apart. Make sure your feet are slightly out so that your calves don't touch the ball.
- Check the natural curves of your spine are present.
- Relax your shoulders and rest your arms by your sides.

Action
Keep your back still as you straighten one knee
- Engage your core by gently drawing your lower abdomen inwards.
- Slowly raise your foot off the ground, straightening your knee to stretch one leg out in front.
- Lower and repeat on the side.
- Do 5 leg raises on each side.

Technique tips
- Keep the ball still and your back straight.
- Breathe normally.

Modifications
- If you find it difficult to maintain a stable position, start with simply raising your heel off the ground, resting your big toe on the floor for balance.
- Progress to lifting your foot just off the floor, keeping your knee bent.
- You can also rest your hands on the ball by your hips for added confidence.

Progressions
- Reaching your arms forward as you raise your leg will further challenge your core.

Seated rotation

Starting position
- Sit tall on a fitball, with your feet out in front, and hip-width apart.
- Check the natural curves of your spine are present and your shoulders are relaxed back and down.
- Relax your shoulders and rest your arms loosely by your sides.

Action
Keep your pelvis still as you turn and reach side to side
- Engage your core and elongate your spine.
- Rotate your upper body side to side, reaching alternate hands past the opposite knee. Keep your legs still while you rotate above the waist.
- Repeat 10 times each side.

Technique tips
- Keep your lower back, pelvis and the ball still.
- Breathe normally and avoid shrugging your shoulders.
- Focus on rotating your upper body rather than reaching with your arms.

Progressions
- Bring your feet and knees together.
- Or raise one leg for 5 rotations, then the other leg.

Mobility, strength and core unite

Fitball wall hover

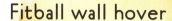

An excellent alternative for women who do not like to be on the floor, horizontal or to take weight through their wrists. This exercise can also be done without a ball, leaning through your forearms on the wall.

Starting position
- Stand with your feet about half a metre away from the wall.
- Hold the ball against the wall at chest height (you should be able to see over the top of the ball).
- Lean forward and rest your forearms on the ball so that your hands are slightly lower than your chin.

Action
Lean through your forearms on the wall
- Elongate your spine, and settle your shoulders down towards your tail bone.
- Visualise your lower abdomen, between your navel and your pubic bone, as you gently draw the area towards your lower back.
- Hold for 5 slow breaths.
- Repeat 3 times.

Technique tips
- Maintain a neutral spine (maintains the natural curves of your back). Do not round your upper back or let your lower back drop into an arch.

Modifications
- Leaning on the wall is less challenging for shoulder girdle stability but is still a great option.

Progressions
- Walk your feet further from the wall.
- If you have no sign of pelvic joint discomfort, you can increase the stability challenge by raising one leg off the floor behind.

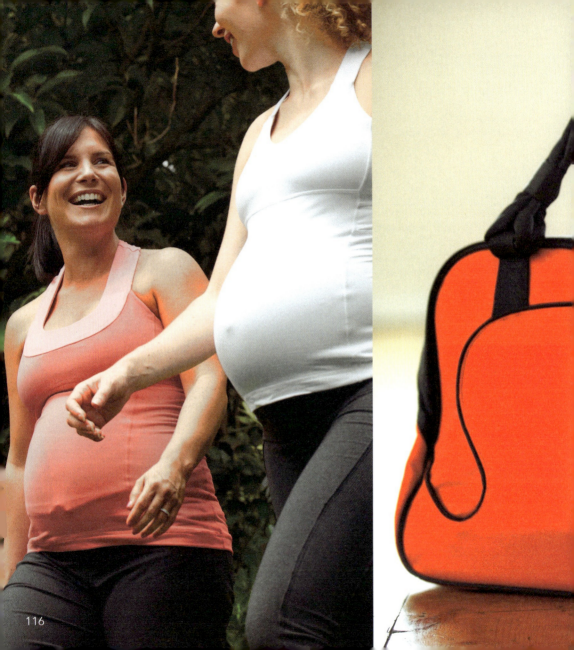

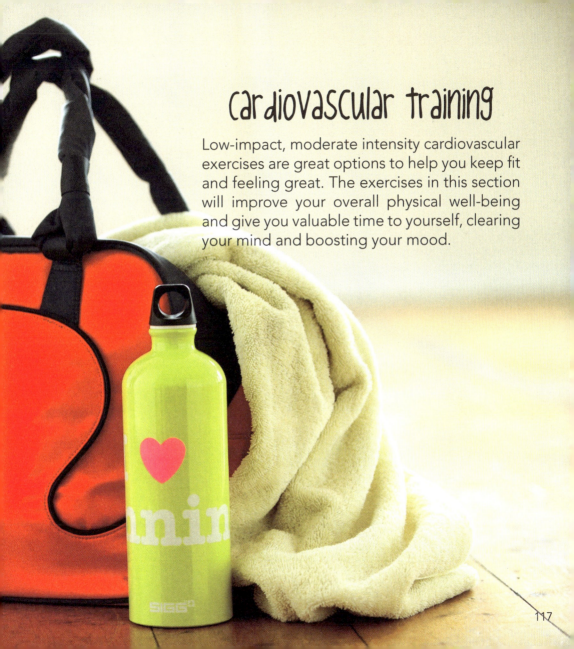

cardiovascular training

Low-impact, moderate intensity cardiovascular exercises are great options to help you keep fit and feeling great. The exercises in this section will improve your overall physical well-being and give you valuable time to yourself, clearing your mind and boosting your mood.

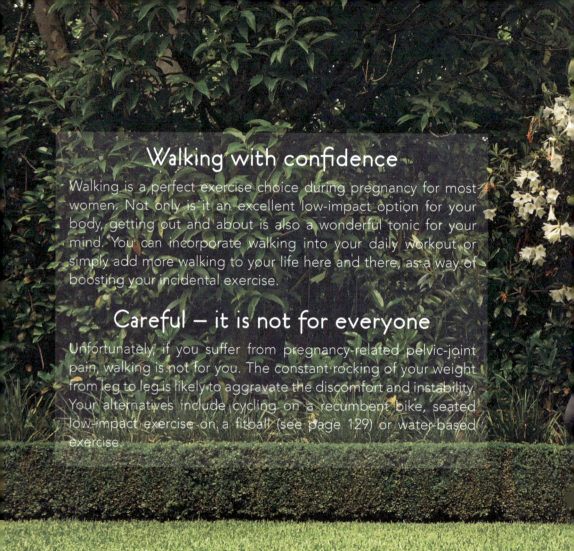

Walking with confidence

Walking is a perfect exercise choice during pregnancy for most women. Not only is it an excellent low-impact option for your body, getting out and about is also a wonderful tonic for your mind. You can incorporate walking into your daily workout, or simply add more walking to your life here and there, as a way of boosting your incidental exercise.

Careful – it is not for everyone

Unfortunately, if you suffer from pregnancy-related pelvic-joint pain, walking is not for you. The constant rocking of your weight from leg to leg is likely to aggravate the discomfort and instability. Your alternatives include cycling on a recumbent bike, seated low-impact exercise on a fitball (see page 129) or water-based exercise.

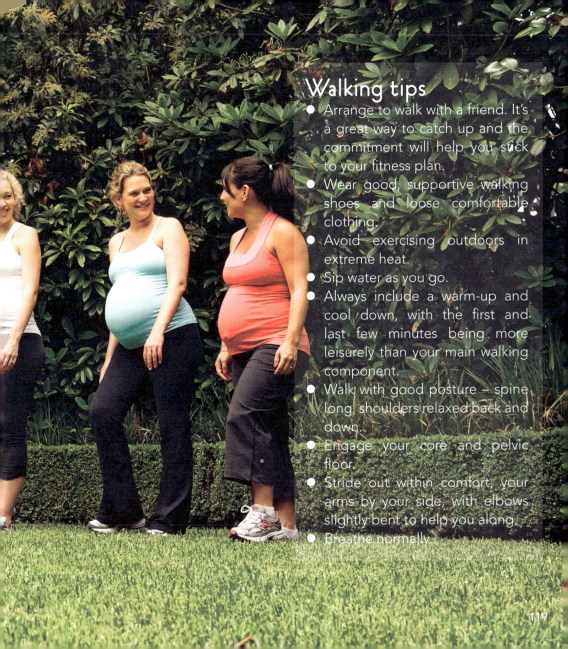

Walking tips

- Arrange to walk with a friend. It's a great way to catch up and the commitment will help you stick to your fitness plan.
- Wear good, supportive walking shoes and loose comfortable clothing.
- Avoid exercising outdoors in extreme heat.
- Sip water as you go.
- Always include a warm-up and cool down, with the first and last few minutes being more leisurely than your main walking component.
- Walk with good posture – spine long, shoulders relaxed back and down.
- Engage your core and pelvic floor.
- Stride out within comfort, your arms by your side, with elbows slightly bent to help you along.
- Breathe normally.

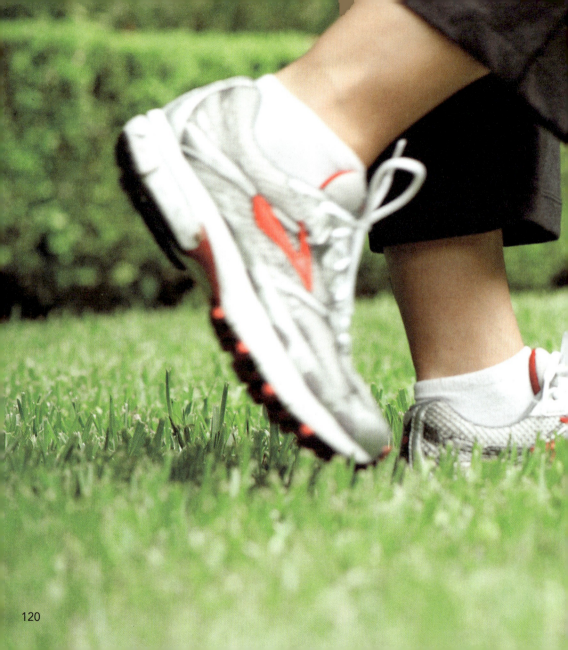

Walking programs

Use your rate of perceived exertion (RPE) to help you choose a walking level that's right for you; 0 is no activity and 20 is working as hard as you possibly could. The most energetic you are advised to work at is 12 to 13. (See 'Listening to your body' page 63).

Level 1 Walking
Ideal for those with minimal prior fitness, especially in the first trimester or if you are wanting to perform light exercise only, at any stage of your pregnancy.

- Walk on a flat, level surface for 2 minutes at a slow stroll, RPE 5.
- If you feel comfortable, pick up your pace to a comfortable walk for 6 minutes, RPE 8.
- Bring it back down to a leisurely stroll for a 2-minute cool down, RPE 5.
- Monitor your body, if this feels too much start with just a few minutes' walk.
- Gradually add 1 minute every few days, within your comfort levels, monitoring your body and energy levels as you go.

Level 2 Walking

You've been walking for a few weeks and feel ready for more, or you were previously fit and well but have been resting the last few weeks and now feel like getting back into activity.

- Walk comfortably on a flat, level surface for 4 minutes, RPE 7.
- Pick up the pace to a brisk walk for 6 to 12 minutes, RPE 10.
- Bring your pace to a stroll for a 4-minute cool down, RPE 7.

Level 3 Walking

You have been exercising moderately prior to your pregnancy and are feeling fit and well.

- Enjoy a comfortable 5-minute warm-up, walking on level or slightly undulating ground, RPE 5.
- Pick up the pace to a slightly faster pace and longer stride, RPE 10.
- Make sure you are engaging your core and pelvic floor and you are not locking your knees.
- Keep your elbows slightly bent, moving naturally by your side.
- Enjoy this 'upbeat walk' for 15 to 30 minutes according to your fitness.
- Bring your pace back to a leisurely stroll for a 5-minute cool down, RPE 5.

Level 4 Walking

Interval training for women who are previously fit and feeling energetic .

- Start with a 5-minute warm-up at a comfortable pace, RPE 7.
- Now increase your pace and energy to a brisker walk, bending your knees, and using your arms more for 5 minutes, RPE 10.
- Pick up your pace to for a 1-minute walk, RPE 12 to13.
- Repeat the cycle alternating 5 minutes at moderate RPE 10 and 1 to 2 minutes of increased energy, RPE 12 to 13.
- Continue for 15 to 30 minutes according to your fitness and how comfortable you are feeling.
- Finish with a 5-minute stroll to cool down, RPE 7.

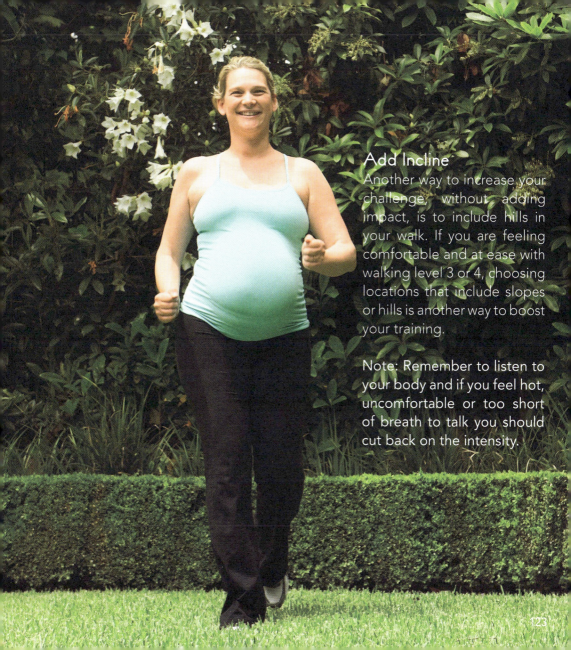

Add Incline
Another way to increase your challenge, without adding impact, is to include hills in your walk. If you are feeling comfortable and at ease with walking level 3 or 4, choosing locations that include slopes or hills is another way to boost your training.

Note: Remember to listen to your body and if you feel hot, uncomfortable or too short of breath to talk you should cut back on the intensity.

Prenatal swimming

A wonderful cardiovascular exercise option, swimming is a no-impact way to boost your fitness during your pregnancy. Being immersed in water provides a welcome respite from the natural heaviness of being pregnant. There are good reasons for pregnant women to exercise in the water: buoyancy, hydrostatic pressure, turbulence and resistance – the water's natural properties – provide a low-stress but highly effective workout that is safe during pregnancy. Many pregnant women express relief as they get into the water, enjoying the lightness and weightless feeling provided by buoyancy, giving your joints, abdomen and pelvis a break from gravity. As your body is immersed in the water, you will also enjoy the benefits of hydrostatic pressure, providing you with all over support which has a similar effect as wearing a total body pressure support stocking. This moves fluid out of your tissues and back into your blood vessels, so helps to reduce swelling (oedema) in your lower limbs, and alleviate the discomfort of varicose veins.

Prenatal swimming basics

Before you start – know your limits

Whatever your prior fitness when exercising in water you must maintain sensible exercise levels, following the general exercise guidelines. If you were a swimmer prior to your pregnancy, it is fine to continue. If you have been exercising energetically on land pre-pregnancy, you may find swimming or aqua exercise a good alternative. You can do more in the pool than on land, thanks to the support, cooling effect and no-impact

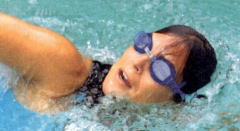

nature of water. If you have been fairly inactive but are comfortable in the water and can swim safely, swimming is a great option for you too. Start with a just a few laps, swimming or walking, and gradually build up your fitness level.

Laps – don't overdo it
Swimming in cool water is a fabulous alternative to other exercises on a hot day. If you are doing laps, be careful not to overdo it. A simple gauge is to make sure you can talk at the end of each lap. Check that you are not overheating. If the pool is cool, this will not be an issue.

Heated pools – stay cool
As a rule, whether swimming or performing other water-based exercise, the ideal pool temperature for pregnant women exercising is 28 degrees or less; you should avoid doing anything more than relaxation and gentle stretches in heated environments such as hydrotherapy pools.

Pelvic-joint pain – no breaststroke kick
Swimming is a fabulous option for women with joint pain, as the buoyancy allows you to exercise without the load of gravity on the joints. If you have

pelvic-joint pain, however, you should modify your swim kick and while breaststroke arms are fine, you must definitely avoid breaststroke leg movements.

Blood pressure – take it easy

Soon after getting into the pool the hydrostatic pressure causes more fluid to go to your kidneys, making some women feel the need to go to the toilet (immersion diuresis). If this happens to you, take your time making your way to the toilet. Always take care when you get out of the pool; leaving the water is similar to removing the pressure support stocking. If you get out quickly, the hydrostatic support is removed suddenly without allowing your body to adjust. To avoid a sudden drop in your blood pressure and dizziness, always make your way to the shallow end of the pool, giving your body a few minutes to get used to less hydrostatic support. Then, slowly leave the water, sitting for a moment on the step or edge before you stand up. If you do experience light-headedness, a cool shower will also help.

Reflux and indigestion – try aqua instead

If you experience reflux or indigestion from being horizontal when swimming you may prefer to perform upright aqua exercises as on pages 176–179.

Swimming guidelines

- Be sure your swimming technique is safe and correct.
- Freestyle and breaststroke are your best styles.
- Kicking with a kickboard is also fine but keep your kicks small and controlled.
- Avoid breaststroke kick if you have pelvic-joint pain.
- Enjoy continuing your pre-pregnancy swimming.
- Start gently if you have been inactive or you are new to swimming.
- Even though you are in water you still need to consider hydration, making sure you sip on water before, during and after your workout.
- Choose upright aqua exercise over swimming if the horizontal position aggravates your reflux or heartburn.
- Try other water-based exercise for effective training and exercise variety (pages 176–179).
- Always get out of the pool slowly and carefully to avoid a sudden drop in blood pressure.
- If you are in doubt about your technique, advice from a swimming teacher will help you get the most out of your time in the pool and help avoid aches and pains related to poor swimming style.
- Do not use the pool if you are having contractions, or experiencing any bleeding, open skin areas, cuts or abrasions, thrush or urinary tract infection.

Swimming programs

Level 1 – You have not been exercising prior to pregnancy

Firstly, make sure you are safe and at ease in the pool and check you have a sound swimming technique. Start with 10 minutes, swimming as far as you feel comfortable, stopping and taking a breather then continuing. Gradually you will be able to increase your time in the pool and distances between rest breaks. You may like to add walking in the water as a part of your water workout to mix things up and keep exercise interesting.

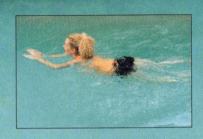

Level 2 – You have been exercising, but not swimming, prior to pregnancy

Even if you have been exercising, it is still important to take it easy when you commence a new exercise style and to check your swimming form. Start with 10 to 15 minutes swimming, resting when you feel short of breath or tired. Gradually build up to 30 minutes.

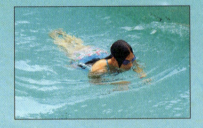

Level 3 – You were swimming prior to pregnancy

If all is well with your pregnancy you can continue swimming within the guidelines of sensible exercise intensity. Modify your style or stroke choice if you notice any discomfort such as pelvic-joint pain. As a time gauge, 30 to 45 minutes is plenty for a pregnancy pool session.

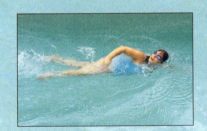

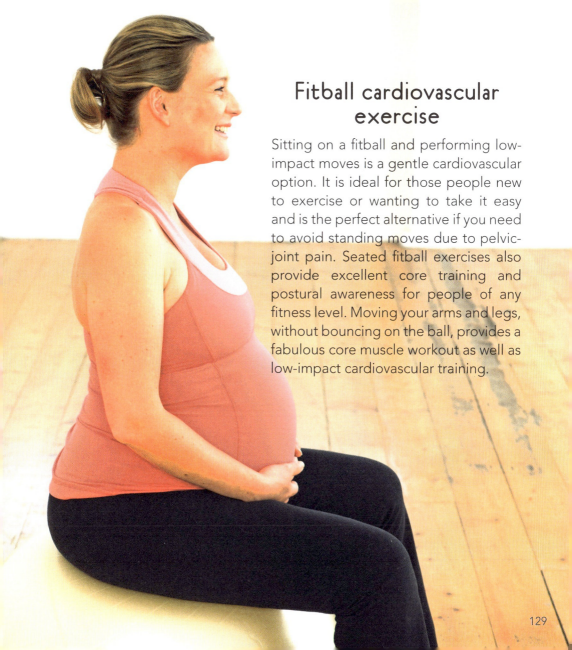

Fitball cardiovascular exercise

Sitting on a fitball and performing low-impact moves is a gentle cardiovascular option. It is ideal for those people new to exercise or wanting to take it easy and is the perfect alternative if you need to avoid standing moves due to pelvic-joint pain. Seated fitball exercises also provide excellent core training and postural awareness for people of any fitness level. Moving your arms and legs, without bouncing on the ball, provides a fabulous core muscle workout as well as low-impact cardiovascular training.

Fitball basics

- You should purchase a burst-resistant quality, correctly sized ball. These are a little more expensive but much safer.
- Inflate your ball to the point of firmness with a little give – not too hard and not too squishy.
- When you sit on the ball, it is the right size if your hips are level with or slightly higher than your knees.
- Make sure you are on a non-slip surface or yoga mat.
- Avoid sharp objects and hot surfaces near the ball.
- Check your posture and form on the ball at all times.
- When you sit on the ball have your feet a little forward so your calves are not touching the ball.
- Sit tall and relax your shoulders down.
- Your lower back should maintain a natural lumbar curve, rather than being flat.
- When performing seated low-impact exercises on the ball resist the temptation to bounce. The more controlled the better the core training as well as less stress on your pelvic floor and uterus.

Gentle low-impact cardiovascular and core training unite

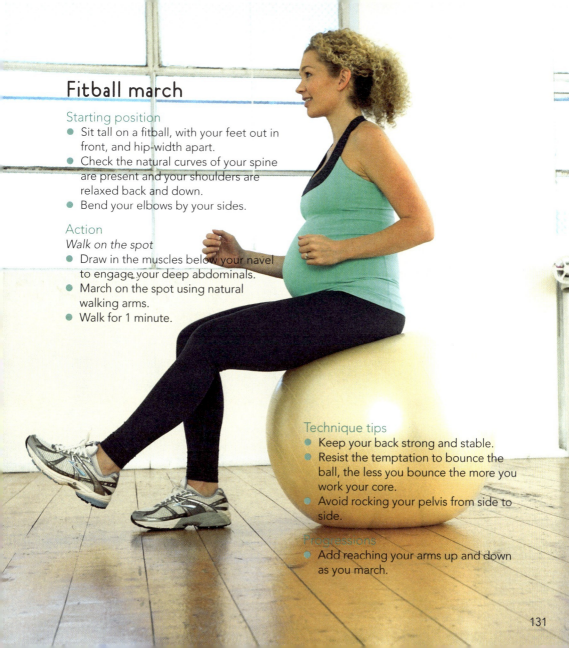

Fitball march

Starting position
- Sit tall on a fitball, with your feet out in front, and hip-width apart.
- Check the natural curves of your spine are present and your shoulders are relaxed back and down.
- Bend your elbows by your sides.

Action
Walk on the spot
- Draw in the muscles below your navel to engage your deep abdominals.
- March on the spot using natural walking arms.
- Walk for 1 minute.

Technique tips
- Keep your back strong and stable.
- Resist the temptation to bounce the ball, the less you bounce the more you work your core.
- Avoid rocking your pelvis from side to side.

Progressions
- Add reaching your arms up and down as you march.

Fitball heel digs

Starting position
- Sit tall on a fitball, with your feet out in front, and hip-width apart.
- Check the natural curves of your spine are present and your shoulders are relaxed back and down.
- Bend your elbows by your sides.

Action
Alternating heel taps
- Draw in the muscles below your navel to engage your deep abdominals.
- Tap alternating heels forward as you reach your arms forward and back.
- Repeat exercise for 1 minute.

Technique tips
- Keep your back strong and stable.
- Resist the temptation to bounce the ball, the less you bounce the more you work your core.
- Bend your elbows back and in as your arms draw backwards.

Progressions
- Slowly raise alternating heels off the ground in front rather than tapping it to the floor.

Seated step touch

Starting position
- Sit tall on a fitball, with your feet out in front and hip-width apart.
- Lengthen your spine and relax your shoulders.

Action
Side step
- Draw in the muscles below your navel to engage your deep abdominals.
- Step your right foot out to the side, then step your left foot across to join it.
- Repeat the step back to the left.
- Continue stepping from side to side.
- Repeat for 1 minute.

Technique tips
- Keep your back strong and stable.
- Resist the temptation to bounce the ball, the less you bounce the more you work your core.

Extra care
- Keep the side step small if you have pelvic-joint discomfort.

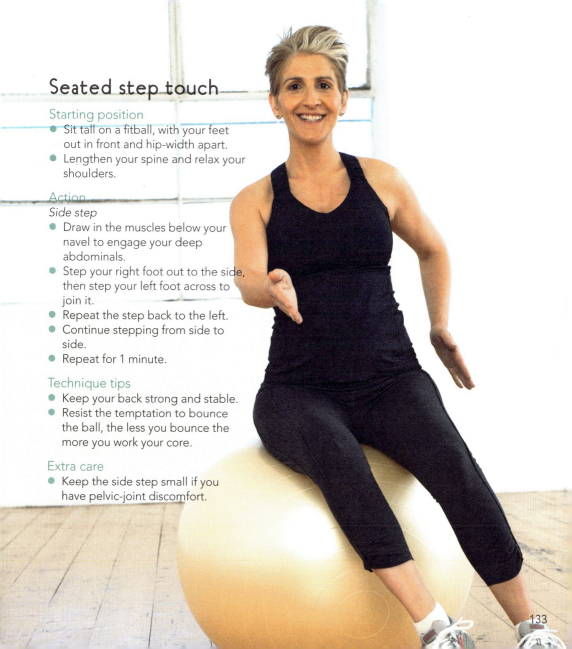

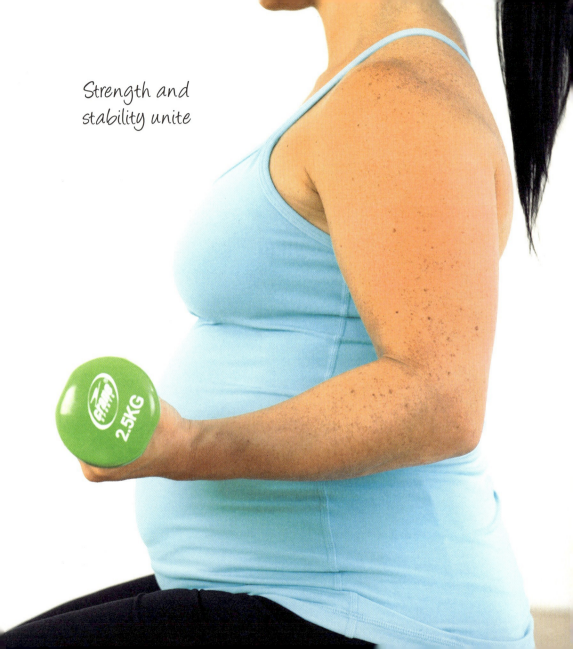

Strength and stability unite

Strength exercises

Strength training is an important component in anyone's fitness program. During your pregnancy sensible muscle conditioning helps you to keep your body toned and strong, helping you and your baby cope with the physical demands of carrying your baby in utero and everyday life.

A sound prenatal strength program has many benefits. Working outer muscles such as those in your arms and legs, maintains muscle strength and definition. Adding focus on muscles specifically important during pregnancy helps your body to support your baby and pregnancy as well as prepare for the physical demands of labour and early motherhood.

Muscle conditioning also assists healthy weight management and, needless to say, a strong body will be more ready to recover after delivery. The vital consideration regarding strength training is to remember that overload and poor technique can cause problems. If you are holding your breath, shaking, or are unable to maintain good posture and stability then you need to decrease the resistance or number of repetitions. Always check you have smooth technique, sound postural control and that you breathe throughout the exercise.

If you have been doing weight training prior to pregnancy, you will be able to continue, but will find you need to lighten the load a little and modify certain exercises such as lying supine after 16 weeks, abdominal curls, and those that stress the pelvis such as lunges, wide squats and single-leg weight-bearing exercises.

Remember your core and pelvic floor

Remember the most important element of strength exercises is sound underlying support from your core and pelvic floor. Always engage your deep abdominals and pelvic floor prior to the exercises. You should be able to maintain this core contraction throughout the exercise.

Signs of top quality strength training

- You are working your core and outer muscles in harmony.
- You breathe naturally throughout the whole exercise.
- You have smooth, controlled technique.
- You balance your training to work opposing muscles equally, e.g. triceps as well as biceps.
- You are keeping other body parts strong and stable; for example, when doing a bicep curl your back should not sway.
- You do not need to use a valsalva (breath holding) technique.

Equipment

There are several muscle conditioning exercises you can perform without any equipment. Some of the following strength exercises incorporate fitballs, hand weights and exercise bands which you can purchase from any sports store. Non-equipment alternatives are provided. A can of tinned food can double up as light hand weights if you prefer. If you have carpal tunnel syndrome with associated weakness then you should not use weights.

Resistance bands are available in light, medium and strong, and are colour coded. You can also shorten them to increase the resistance by wrapping them around your hand one more time. Some come as simple straps, others have handles. For fitball information, see 'Fitball cardiovascular exercise' (pages 129–133).

Modify your load and repetitions for perfect form and control

Your strength dictates how heavy your resistance should be. You should be feeling your muscles work during the last few repetitions of a set, but still able to maintain sound technique. If you feel like you could do another 20 repetitions you need heavier weights and if you can not maintain good form and finish the set, you need to lighten your load or perform a few less repetitions.

	Resistance guide			
	Just starting exercise. Previously inactive	Feeling strong but no formal weights work recently	Have been working with weights up until pregnancy, but nothing for a few weeks or months	Have been working with weights prior to and during pregnancy
Weights	0.5 – 1 kg	1 – 3 kg	1 – 3 kg	3 – 4 kg
Resistance band	Light	Light – medium	Light – medium	Medium – strong

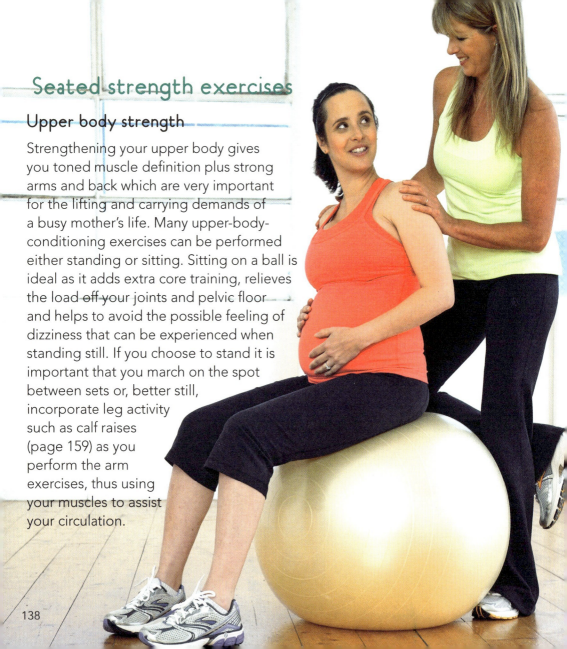

Seated strength exercises

Upper body strength

Strengthening your upper body gives you toned muscle definition plus strong arms and back which are very important for the lifting and carrying demands of a busy mother's life. Many upper-body-conditioning exercises can be performed either standing or sitting. Sitting on a ball is ideal as it adds extra core training, relieves the load off your joints and pelvic floor and helps to avoid the possible feeling of dizziness that can be experienced when standing still. If you choose to stand it is important that you march on the spot between sets or, better still, incorporate leg activity such as calf raises (page 159) as you perform the arm exercises, thus using your muscles to assist your circulation.

Lateral raise

Starting position
- Sitting tall on the fitball, on a bench, or standing.
- Hold your weights by your sides.
- Elbows bent to 90 degrees.
- Shoulders relaxed back and down.

Action
Side raise
- Raise your arms sideways until your hands and elbows are level with your shoulders.
- Lower your arms slowly.
- 15 repetitions x 2 sets.

Technique tips
- Avoid tensing your neck or shoulder muscles.
- As you raise your arms draw your shoulder blades back and down.

Modifications
- Decrease the size of weights.

Progressions
- Increase your weights.
- If sitting on a ball, add an alternating leg raise.

Extra care
- Perform without hand weights if you have carpal tunnel syndrome.

Low row

Starting position
- Sitting tall on a fitball, or standing.
- Feet hip-width apart.
- Holding hand weights, thumbs up.
- Elbows bent and tucked in by your sides.
- Shoulders drawing back and down.

Action
Row
- Reach forward to extend your arms in front to waist height.
- Draw your elbows backwards bringing the weights back towards your hips.
- 15 repetitions x 2 sets.

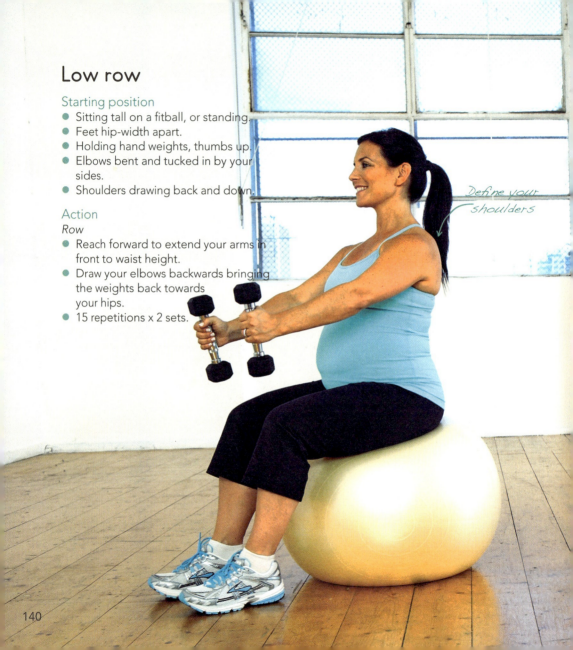

Define your shoulders

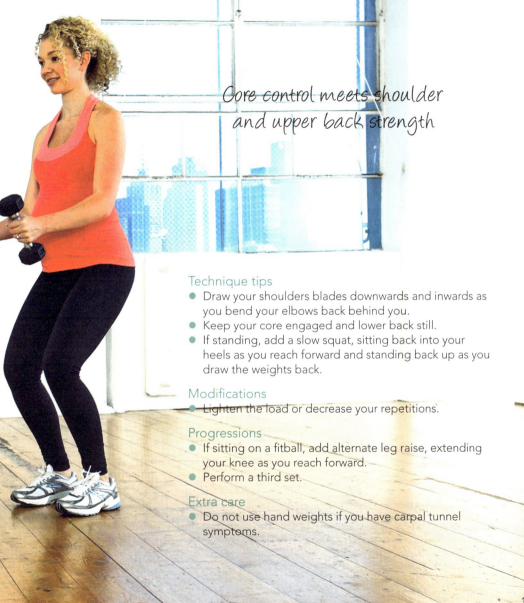

Core control meets shoulder and upper back strength

Technique tips
- Draw your shoulders blades downwards and inwards as you bend your elbows back behind you.
- Keep your core engaged and lower back still.
- If standing, add a slow squat, sitting back into your heels as you reach forward and standing back up as you draw the weights back.

Modifications
- Lighten the load or decrease your repetitions.

Progressions
- If sitting on a fitball, add alternate leg raise, extending your knee as you reach forward.
- Perform a third set.

Extra care
- Do not use hand weights if you have carpal tunnel symptoms.

Bicep curl

Starting position
- Sitting tall on a fitball or bench, or standing.
- Feet hip-width apart.
- Holding hand weights by your side, palms facing forwards.
- Shoulders drawing back and down.

Action
Bend and straighten
- Slowly bend your elbows bringing your weights up towards your shoulders.
- Lower them back down with control.
- 15 repetitions x 2 sets.

Technique tips
- Keep your elbows tucked in by your sides and your upper arms still.
- If standing, add a slow squat, sitting back and down as you bend your elbows.

Modifications
- Lighten the load or decrease your repetitions.

Progressions
- If sitting on a fitball, add alternate leg raise, extending your knee as you bend your elbows.
- Increase your load or add a third set.

Extra care
- Do not use hand weights if you have carpal tunnel symptoms.

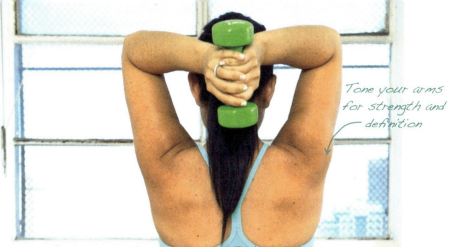

Tone your arms for strength and definition

Triceps press

Starting position
- Sitting tall on a fitball or standing.
- Holding one weight in both hands with your arms raised and elbows bent so the weight is behind your head.
- Shoulders drawing downwards and elbows tucked in close to your head.

Action
Press to the sky
- Engage your core, gently hugging your baby with your deep abdominals.
- Extend your elbows pushing your hand weight upwards.
- Bend your elbows to lower the weight back to behind your head.
- 15 repetitions x 2 sets.

Technique tips
- You may use one heavy weight or two light to medium weights.
- Push the weight upwards not forwards.
- Check your posture and do not let your back sway.
- If standing add a calf raise between each triceps press.

Modifications
- Lighten the load.
- Perform 10 repetitions x 2 sets.

Progressions
- If sitting on the ball add alternating leg raises for extra core challenge.
- Add an extra set.

Extra care
- Exercises with arms raised high involve extra core control, so focus on your core and stop this exercise if you experience lower back discomfort or inability to stabilise.

External rotation

Starting position
- Sitting tall on a fitball, on a bench, or standing.
- Hold a resistance band between your hands.
- Arms by your sides, elbows bent to 90 degrees.
- Shoulders drawing back and down.

Action
- Rotate one shoulder to stretch the band outwards to one side, while holding it still with the stabilising arm.
- Repeat x 10 then change to the other side.
- 10 repetitions on each side x 2 sets.

Technique tips
- Keep your elbow tucked in close and in contact with your side.

Modifications
- You can perform this exercise with light weights or no equipment.

Progressions
- Open both arms at the same time.
- Add a single leg raise, holding your right leg up while you work your right arm and the left leg up whilst you work the left arm.

Seated semi-squat

Starting position
- Sit a little forward on a ball or chair, with your fingers resting by hips.
- Feet out in front of the ball, hip-width apart.
- Elongate your spine and settle your shoulders downwards.

Action
Start to stand then sit back down
- Lean slightly forward to take your weight into your heels.
- Raise your bottom just off the ball then slowly sit back down. Keep your fingers in contact with the ball, standing only as high as your arm length allows.
- 15 repetitions x 3 sets.

Technique tips
- It is very important you keep both hands in contact with the ball. This ensures you stay straight and stops the ball from rolling away.
- Keep your back straight and head up, Imagine you have a jug of water on your head and you don't want any water to spill.

Modifications
- Raise only slightly keeping your bottom in contact with the ball.

Progressions
- Increase repetitions to 20 per set.

Extra care
- If you find your knees are uncomfortable or if you prefer a gentler exercise, replace with seated leg raise (page 113).

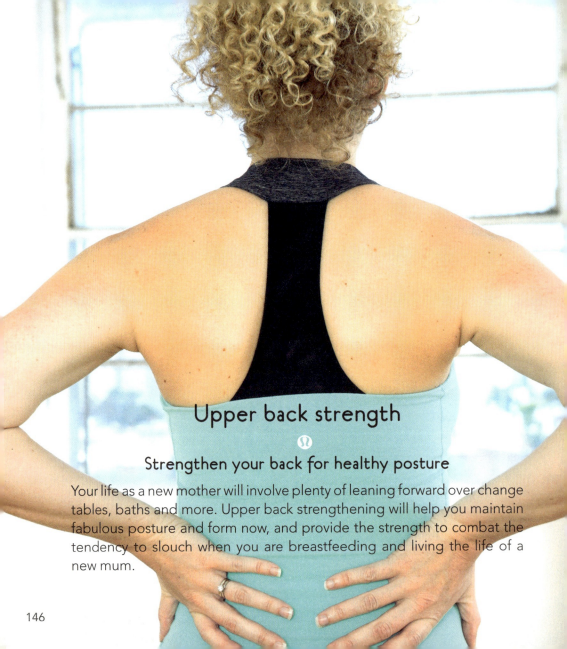

Upper back strength

Strengthen your back for healthy posture

Your life as a new mother will involve plenty of leaning forward over change tables, baths and more. Upper back strengthening will help you maintain fabulous posture and form now, and provide the strength to combat the tendency to slouch when you are breastfeeding and living the life of a new mum.

Lat pull down

Starting position
- Sitting or standing tall.
- Your arms are reaching up and angled slightly forward, hands holding a resistance band, shoulder-width apart.
- Engage your core and settle your shoulder blades downwards.

Action
Pull wide
- Slowly bend your elbows down and back, drawing your hands down and out wide to stretch the band.
- Feel the muscles in your back work as though you are trying to close a heavy window.
- Slowly release the tension, raising your hands up and inwards.
- 15 repetitions x 2 sets.

Technique tips
- Start with the band on slight tension.
- Take your hands wider than your elbows as you stretch the band out and downwards.
- Use your core abdominals and make sure your back does not sway.
- If you are standing add slow squats and walk on the spot between sets.

Modifications
- Perform the exercise without a band using a strong controlled technique so that you still feel the muscles in your back working.
- Perform 10 repetitions x 2 sets.

Progressions
- Add alternating leg extensions for added core challenge.
- Slightly shorten the band.

Extra care
- Exercises involving arms raised above your head involve extra core control, so leave them out if you experience lower back discomfort or inability to stabilise in this position.

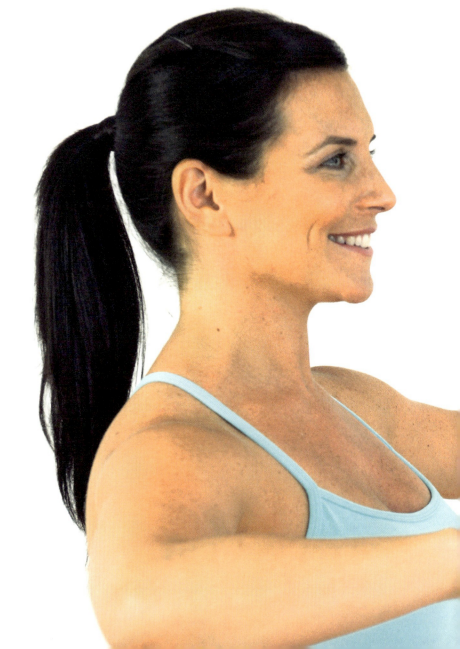

Wide row

Starting position
- Sitting tall on a fitball or bench, or standing.
- Hold a resistance band out in front of you at chest height, palms facing downwards and a shoulder-width apart.
- Engage your core and settle your shoulders back and down.

Action
Bend your elbows and stretch the band wide
- Slowly bend your elbows and draw your hands wide to stretch the band.
- Feel the muscles between your shoulder blades creating the action.
- Release the tension carefully, bringing your hands back to the front.
- 15 repetitions x 2 sets.

Technique tips
- Start with the band on slight tension.
- Take your hands wider than your elbows as you draw them outwards and backwards.
- If standing perform calf raises or squats as you extend the band.

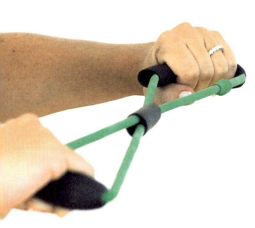

Modifications
- Perform the exercise without a band using a strong controlled technique so that you still feel the muscles between your shoulder blades working.
- Lengthen the band slightly.
- Perform 10 repetitions x 2 sets.

Progressions
- Add alternating leg extensions for added core challenge.
- Slightly shorten the band.

Four-point kneeling

An excellent position for strengthening your core muscles, back, arms and shoulders simultaneously. As well as alleviating the heavy load off your pelvis, the action of gravity on your growing abdomen provides some resistance to help you train your core abdominals.

Triceps kick back

Starting position
- Kneeling on all fours, with your hands under shoulders and knees under hips.
- Soften your elbows, drawing your shoulders towards your tail bone.
- Elongate your spine and keep your back straight while still maintaining the natural curve in your back. Look down at the floor to keep your neck in line with your spine.
- Move to a 3-point kneeling position by taking a hand weight in your right hand, bending your elbow, tucking it in by your side.

Action
Triceps press
- Engage your core muscles, gently hugging your baby towards your spine with your deep abdominals.
- Straighten your elbow to push the hand weight to your hip, then slowly bend it back again.
- Perform 15, then rest back on your heels before resuming the kneeling position and repeating with your left arm.
- 15 repetition x 2 sets.

Technique tips
- Keep your core engaged and breathe normally throughout the exercise.
- Keep your upper arm still, high and tucked in close your side.

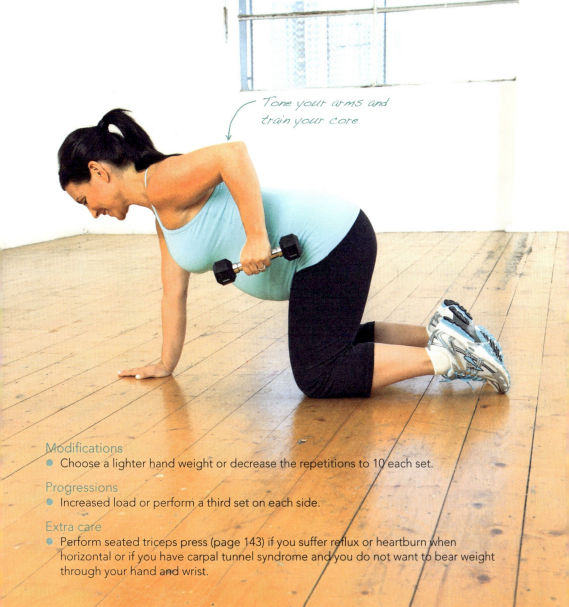

Tone your arms and train your core

Modifications
- Choose a lighter hand weight or decrease the repetitions to 10 each set.

Progressions
- Increased load or perform a third set on each side.

Extra care
- Perform seated triceps press (page 143) if you suffer reflux or heartburn when horizontal or if you have carpal tunnel syndrome and you do not want to bear weight through your hand and wrist.

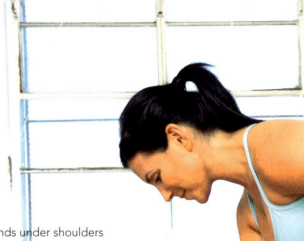

Kneeling push back

Starting position
- Kneeling on all fours, with your hands under shoulders and knees under hips.
- Soften your elbows, drawing your shoulders towards your tail bone.
- Elongate your spine and keep your back straight while still maintaining the natural curve in your back. Look down at the floor to keep your neck in line with your spine.
- Move to a 3-point kneeling position by taking a hand weight in your right hand, holding it just off the floor.

Action
Lateral push back
- Keeping your elbow slightly bent, raise your arm to your side. Slowly lower your arm.
- Perform 15, then rest back on your heels before resuming the kneeling position and repeating with your left arm.
- 15 repetition x 2 sets.

Technique tips
- Look at the floor and keep your neck in line with your spine.
- Engage your core muscles and maintain a straight strong back.

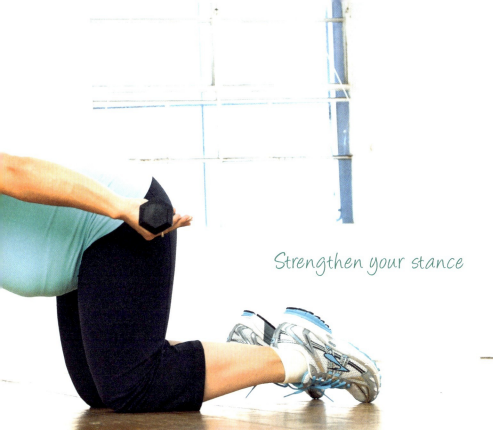

Strengthen your stance

Modifications
- Choose a lighter hand weight or decrease the repetitions to 10 each set.

Progressions
- Increased load or perform a third set on each side.

Extra care
- Perform seated lateral pull down (page 147) if you suffer reflux or heartburn, if you have carpal tunnel syndrome and do not want to bear weight through your hand and wrist or if you have trouble getting down and up off the floor.

Kneeling single arm row

Starting position
- Kneeling on all fours, with your hands under shoulders and knees under hips.
- Soften your elbows, drawing your shoulders towards your tail bone.
- Elongate your spine and keep your back straight while still maintaining the natural curve in your back. Look down at the floor to keep your neck in line with your spine.
- Move to a 3-point kneeling position by taking a hand weight.

Action
Bend your arm up and outward
- Engage your core muscles, gently hugging your baby towards your spine with your deep abdominals.
- Raise your right arm sideways, level with your shoulder.
- Take your hand out wider than your elbow as you focus on drawing your right shoulder blade inwards.
- Perform 15 then rest back on your heels to rest, or perform a pelvic-floor lift before resuming the kneeling position and repeating with your left arm.
- 15 repetitions x 2 sets.

Technique tip
- Look at the floor and keep your neck in line with your spine.

Modifications
- Choose a lighter hand weight or decrease the repetitions to 10 each set.

Progressions
- Increased load or perform a third set on each side.

Extra care
- Replace with seated wide row (page 149) if you do not like to lean through your wrists or be in horizontal positions due to reflux or heartburn.

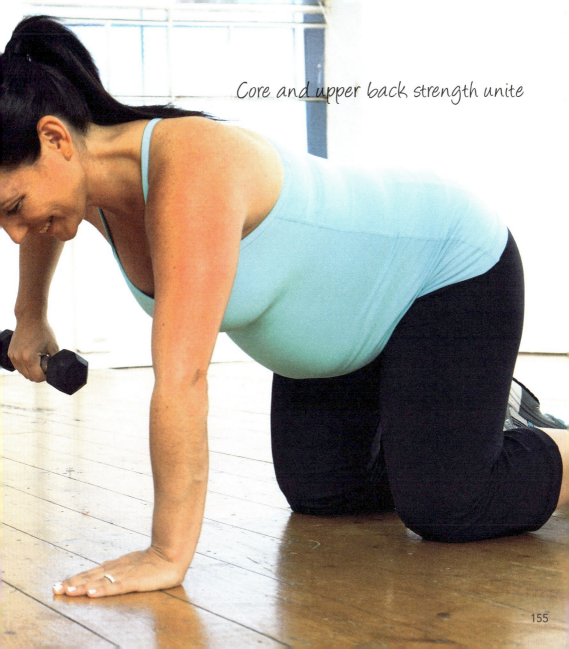

Core and upper back strength unite

Kneeling abdominal curl

Although it is not recommended that you strain your abdominals with supine abdominal curls, it is still a good idea to gently exercises your outer abdominals to remind them that they exist.

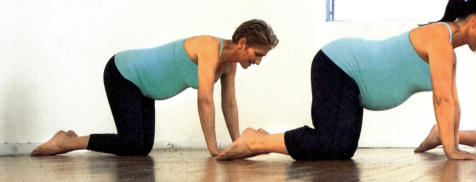

Starting position
- Kneeling on all fours, with your hands under shoulders and knees under hips.
- Soften your elbows, drawing your shoulders towards your tail bone.
- Elongate your spine and keep your back straight while still maintaining the natural curve in your back. Look down at the floor to keep your neck in line with your spine.

Action
Engage your abs to round your back
- Take your focus to your outer abdominals running from your rib cage to your pelvis.
- Engage your core abdominals by drawing your lower abdomen towards your lower back.
- Now switch on those outer abdominal muscles to bring your pelvis towards your rib cage, rounding your back.
- Release slowly to lower back to the starting position.
- 10 repetitions.

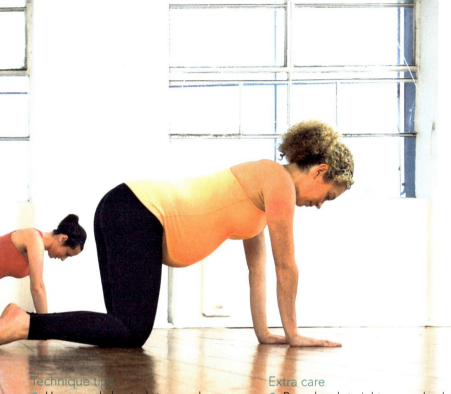

Technique tips
- Use your abdominals to round your back. It is easy to slip into the habit of using the muscles of your arms and legs to do this instead.

Modifications
- Sitting on a fitball is a gentle way to round and straighten your back.

Extra care
- Round and straighten your back in the same way, sitting on a fitball or standing, if you do not like to be on your hands and knees.

Kneel and lean

Common abdominal exercises, such as the plank (where you have a straight body propped on your forearms and toes) place too much stress on the pregnant back. A great alternative is leaning gently forward on a fitball. You work the same muscles but with less stress.

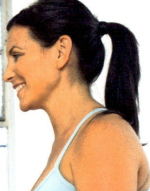

Starting position
- Kneel upright with the fitball in front of you and reach your arms out to rest on the top of the ball.
- Draw your shoulders back and down.
- Engage your core muscles, gently hugging your baby towards your spine with your deep abdominals.
- Maintain straight posture from shoulders to knees.

Action
Lean forward
- Bend your elbows as you lean forward, keeping them tucked in close to your sides.
- Keep your shoulders down and your upper back straight throughout the exercise.
- Use your core muscles to support your lower back.
- Keep your hips straight.
- Hold for 5 slow breaths, then return to the starting position.
- Repeat 3 times.

Technique tips
- Keep your back straight.
- Do not allow your back to sway or your hips to bend.

Modifications
- Fitball wall hover or wall lean and reach on page 115.
- Seated leg raise on page 113.

Progressions
- Roll the ball a little further forward to increase the stability challenge.

Extra care
- The fitball wall hover may be preferable if you do not like to lean through your hands or get down on the floor.

Standing strength

The following exercises include some effective ways to strengthen and tone your calves, thighs and gluteals, plus an excellent wall push up alternative. This is much safer than the usual push up, because it is upright it works the same muscles but with less stress on your back and shoulders.

Calf raise

Starting position
- Stand tall with your feet hip-width apart.
- Shoulders drawing back and down.
- Knees soft (slightly bent).

Action
Raise up and down
- Lift your pelvic floor and engage your core.
- Roll your weight forward into the balls of your feet.
- Raise your heels slowly up off the floor and then slowly down to lift and lower your body.
- 15 repetitions x 3 sets.

Technique tips
- Focusing on a spot about 1 metre in front on the floor can help you to keep your balance.

Modifications
- Perform calf raises with a ball between your lower back and the wall.

Progressions
- Add an arm-strengthening move such as lateral raise (page 139).

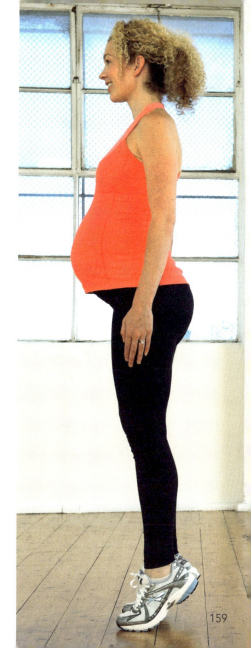

Narrow-based squat

Everyone wants strong thighs. They are particularly useful for women who are expecting. Not only do they look good, but strong leg muscles help you when you are lifting and are vital if you are wanting an active upright labour. A narrow squat is less stressful on your pelvic joints than a wide based squat or lunge.

Starting position
- Stand tall with your feet hip-width apart.
- Shoulders drawing back and down.
- Knees soft (slightly bent).

Action
Stand and squat
- Roll your shoulders back and down, engage your core abdominals.
- Keep your weight in your heels as you sit back and down, bending your knees and hips so that you incline your torso slightly forward and your pelvis backwards.
- Press your heels into the ground as you stand back up, tucking your tail bone in and under at the top.
- Continue with the exercise by slowly repeating the squat.
- 15 repetitions x 3 sets.

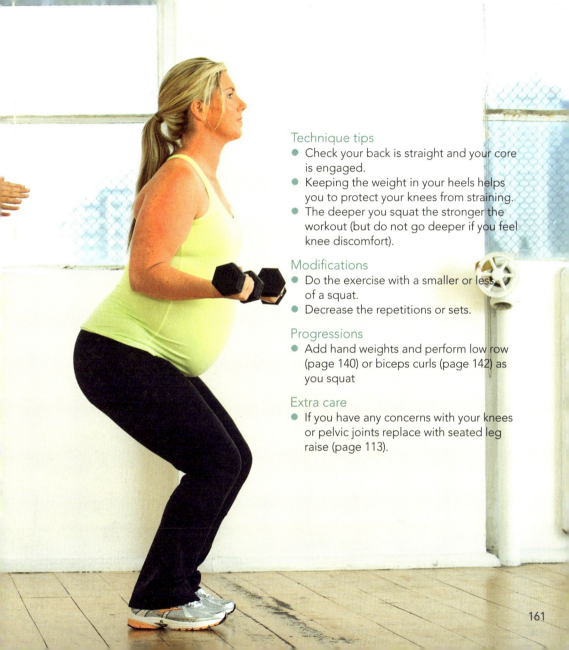

Technique tips
- Check your back is straight and your core is engaged.
- Keeping the weight in your heels helps you to protect your knees from straining.
- The deeper you squat the stronger the workout (but do not go deeper if you feel knee discomfort).

Modifications
- Do the exercise with a smaller or less of a squat.
- Decrease the repetitions or sets.

Progressions
- Add hand weights and perform low row (page 140) or biceps curls (page 142) as you squat

Extra care
- If you have any concerns with your knees or pelvic joints replace with seated leg raise (page 113).

Wall squat

The wall squat is an excellent way to strengthen your thighs. It is different to the regular squat as it allows you to keep your back upright and incorporates extra core conditioning.

Starting position
- Stand with the ball between your lower back and the wall with your feet hip-width apart.
- Slowly roll down into the 'seated position'.
- Adjust your feet, walking them out until you can see your toes beyond your knees.
- Check the ball is supporting your pelvis and lower back at the lowest seated position.
- Your back should be straight and parallel to the wall.

Action
Stand and sit
- Draw your lower abdomen towards the wall, engaging your core.
- Place the weight in your heels and slowly roll the ball up the wall to a standing position. Repeat.
- 15 repetitions x 3 sets.

Technique tips
- Your back should be vertical, do not lean forward or backward.
- Keep your weight in your heels to protect your knees.
- Think of drawing your lower abdomen towards the wall.

Modifications
- Do the exercise with a smaller or less of a squat.
- Decrease the repetitions or sets.

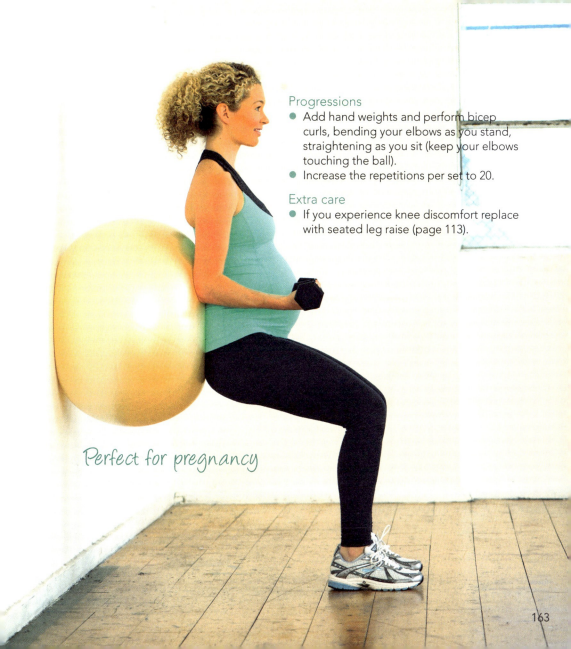

Progressions
- Add hand weights and perform bicep curls, bending your elbows as you stand, straightening as you sit (keep your elbows touching the ball).
- Increase the repetitions per set to 20.

Extra care
- If you experience knee discomfort replace with seated leg raise (page 113).

Perfect for pregnancy

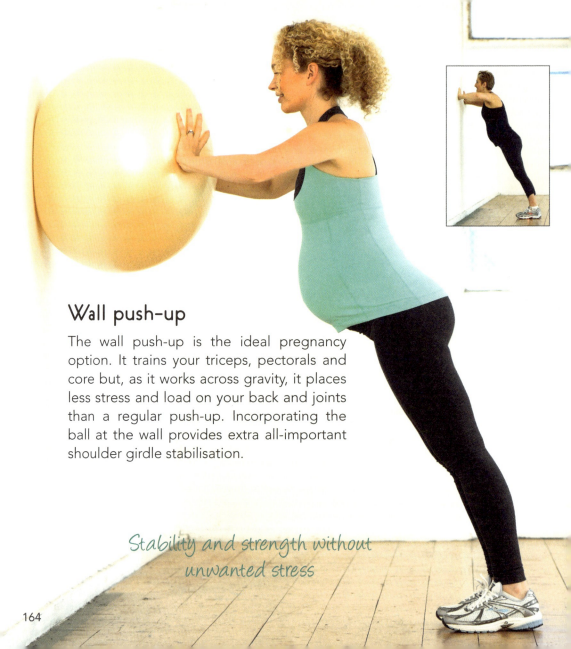

Wall push-up

The wall push-up is the ideal pregnancy option. It trains your triceps, pectorals and core but, as it works across gravity, it places less stress and load on your back and joints than a regular push-up. Incorporating the ball at the wall provides extra all-important shoulder girdle stabilisation.

Stability and strength without unwanted stress

Starting position
- Stand upright with your arms outstretched, holding the ball against the wall at shoulder height.
- Set your shoulders shown to stabilise your shoulder blades and deep abdominals.
- Step back away from the wall.

Action
Upright push-up
- Lightly turn on your buttocks to keep your hips straight.
- Now perform slow push-ups, bending your elbows outwards as you lean towards the wall and straightening them to push away.
- 15 repetitions x 3 sets.

Technique tips
- Keep your shoulder blades down.
- Do not bend at the hips or allow your back to sway or arch.
- You should be able to see over the top of the ball at all times.
- Be careful not to hyperextend your elbows as you push away.

Modifications
- Decrease the repetitions or sets.
- Perform the wall push-up without the ball, with your hands placed shoulder-width apart on the wall at shoulder height.

Progressions
- Walk your feet further away from the wall to increase the workload.
- Increase to 20 repetitions per set.

Extra care
- Replace with fitball wall hover (page 115) if you do not like to lean through your wrists.

Ball bridge

This exercise allows you to work your gluteals against gravity and is an alternative to the regular bridge, which is inappropriate after 16 weeks due to the chance of supine hypotension. The difference is that being on the ball allows you to have your hips lower than your chest and your body at an angle. As long as you do not hold your hips up in the horizontal position you are not maintaining a supine position.

Starting position
- Sit with your hands by your hips on the ball.
- Round your back and slowly walk out as you roll down to place your elbows on the fitball.
- Continue until your shoulder blades are on the ball.
- Now rest your head back on the ball.
- You should be in a straight position, with your head, neck and shoulder girdle on the ball, your back straight and your heels directly under your knees and hip-width apart.

Action
Lower and raise your hips
- Engage your core abdominals by drawing your lower abdomen towards your lower back.
- Place the weight in your heels.
- Slowly lower and raise your hips, using your gluteals (or bottom muscles) to lift your pelvis. Rise to horizontal, as explained above.
- To rest between sets, put your elbows on the ball to keep it underneath you, lower your hips and bring your head off the ball.
- To sit back up, lower your hips, put your elbows on the ball and lift your head off the ball. Now put your chin on your chest as you walk back and the ball will 'roll you up'. It is important to send your head forward.
- 10 to 15 repetitions x 2 sets.

Work your butt and back

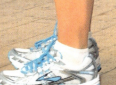

Technique tips
- You must engage your core muscles.
- Your neck should be in line with your spine and the ball should be supporting your head, neck and shoulder blades.
- If your chin is on your chest, roll back a little on the ball.
- Pushing your heels into the ground and focusing on using your gluteal muscles improves the quality of the exercise.

Modifications
- Decrease the number of repetitions or sets.
- If you don't feel comfortable doing this exercise replace it with a seated leg raise or wall squat (pages 162–163).

Progressions
- Bring your feet and knees closer together.

Extra care
- If you feel back discomfort try improving your core muscle recruitment. If you continue to feel lower back discomfort, then replace with seated leg raise (page 113).

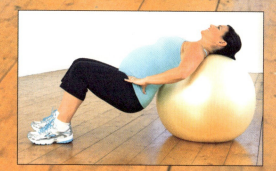

Lying on the floor strength

Lying on your side on the floor is a lovely position for relaxing as well as working your pelvic floor. It is also an option for gluteal and thigh strengthening.

Side leg raise

Starting position
- Lying on your side with your bottom leg bent for stability, relax your neck and shoulders.
- Your top leg must be straight and pointing forward.
- Rest your head on the floor or your hand.
- Breathe normally.

Action
Raise and lower your leg
- Engage your core and straighten your top leg.
- Keeping your foot and knee pointing straight ahead, lift your heel just a little off the floor, then lower to the floor slowly.
- 5 repetitions x 3 sets.

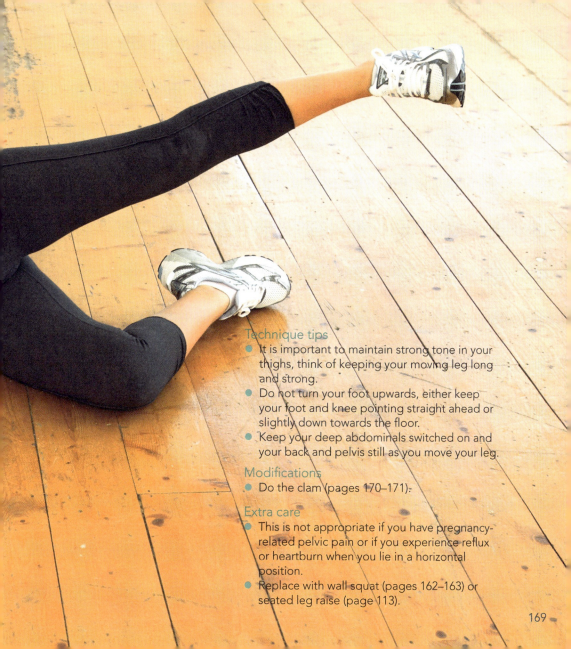

Technique tips
- It is important to maintain strong tone in your thighs, think of keeping your moving leg long and strong.
- Do not turn your foot upwards, either keep your foot and knee pointing straight ahead or slightly down towards the floor.
- Keep your deep abdominals switched on and your back and pelvis still as you move your leg.

Modifications
- Do the clam (pages 170–171).

Extra care
- This is not appropriate if you have pregnancy-related pelvic pain or if you experience reflux or heartburn when you lie in a horizontal position.
- Replace with wall squat (pages 162–163) or seated leg raise (page 113).

Clam

Starting position
- Lie on your side with both knees bent so that your hips and knees are at 90 degrees, knees and feet together.

Action
Open and close your top leg
- Gently draw your lower abdomen inwards to hug your baby with your deep abdominals.
- Keeping your feet together and on the floor, slowly raise and lower your top knee.
- Repeat 10 times.
- Slowly roll over to repeat the clam on the other side, keeping your knees and feet together as you do.

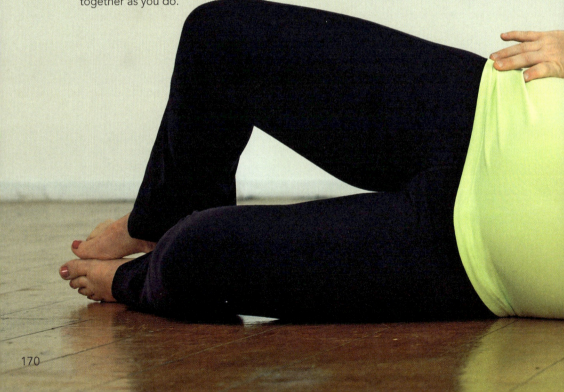

Technique tips
- Breathe normally.
- Relax your head and neck.

Extra care
- Replace with any upright core exercise such as the seated leg raise (page 113) if you suffer reflux or heartburn in horizontal positions.

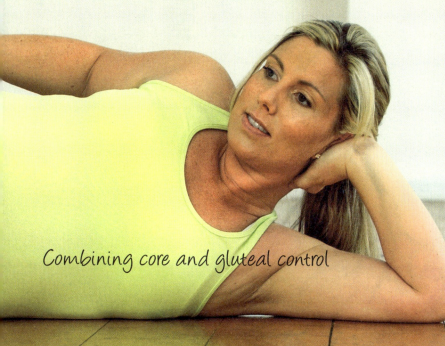

Combining core and gluteal control

Bridging

Starting position
- Lie on your back on the floor, with knees bent and feet on the floor, hip-width apart.
- Relax your arms by your side.
- Relax your neck and shoulders.

Action
Raise and lower your bottom
- Push your heels into the ground and squeeze your gluteals (bottom muscles) as you raise your hips and your lower back off the floor.
- Slowly roll your spine back down to the floor.
- 15 repetitions x 3 sets.

Technique tip
- Keep your core engaged and your arms, neck and shoulders relaxed.

Modification
- Slightly lift your hips off the floor.

Progressions
- Keep your knees and feet together.

Extra care
- This is not appropriate after 16 weeks.
- Replace with the clam (pages 170–171), ball bridge (pages 166–167) or wall squat (pages 162–163) after 16 weeks.

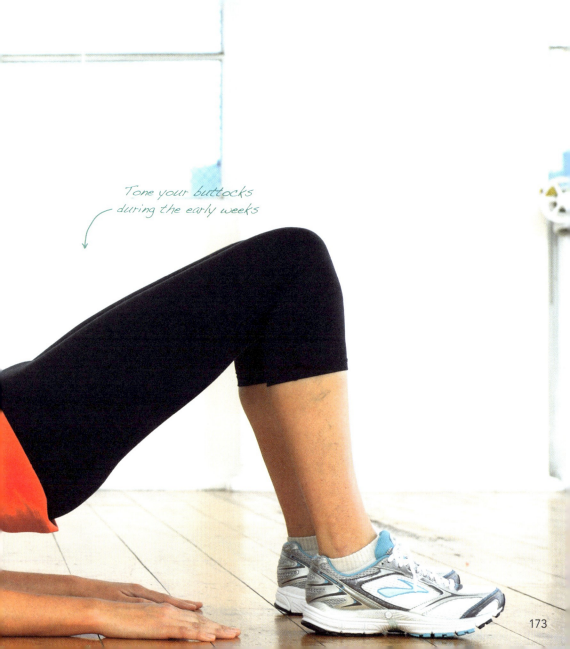

Hamstring lift and roll

An excellent way to strengthen your core, gluteals and hamstrings but appropriate for the first 16 weeks only.

Starting position
- Lie on your back on the floor with your heels resting on top of the ball.
- Relax your arms by your side.
- Relax your neck and shoulders.

Action
Lift and roll
- Gently draw your lower abdomen towards the floor to engage your core.
- Push your heels into the ball as you raise your bottom off the floor.
- Bend your knees and roll the ball slowly towards your body until your knees are bent above your hips.
- Roll the ball away again.
- Gently lower your hips and pelvis back to the floor.
- 10 repetitions x 3 sets.

Technique tips
- Keep your feet flexed back towards you so the back of your heels, not the soles of your feet, are in contact with the ball.

Modifications
- Slightly raise your bottom off the floor.
- If you do not have a ball, replace with Bridges (page 172).

Progressions
- Take your arms off the floor to increase stability challenge, resting them across your chest.

Extra care
- This exercise is appropriate during the first 16 weeks only.

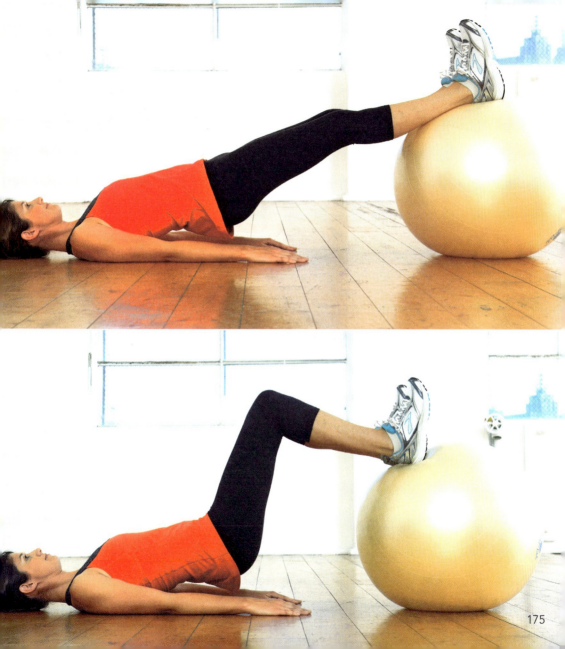

Aqua exercise

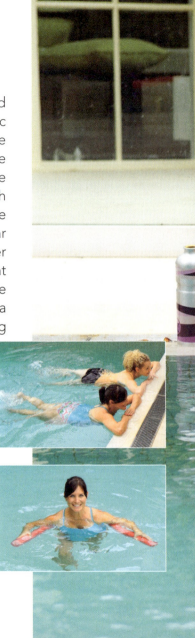

Swimming is just one of the many water-based exercise options. The buoyancy and hydrostatic pressure of water make it an excellent exercise environment for prenatal women. Walking in the water, performing strength moves using the resistance of the water, kicking at the wall, and working with aqua equipment such as noodles opens a whole new world to prenatal fitness. If you attend a regular aqua group exercise class, be sure to work no harder than moderate intensity, and avoid exercises that strain your joints, such as prolonged standing on one leg. Your ideal option is a pregnancy-specific aqua exercise class but you may also like to try the following exercises when you are next in the pool.

At the wall

- Floating on your front at the wall with your hands supporting you on the edge or rail.
- Kick with straight legs for 30 to 60 seconds.
- Rest and repeat 3 times.

Deep water running

- Place a noodle behind your back and under your arms to help you float.
- Lift your feet off the pool floor.
- Work your legs in a running action, keeping your core and pelvic floor engaged and your back straight.

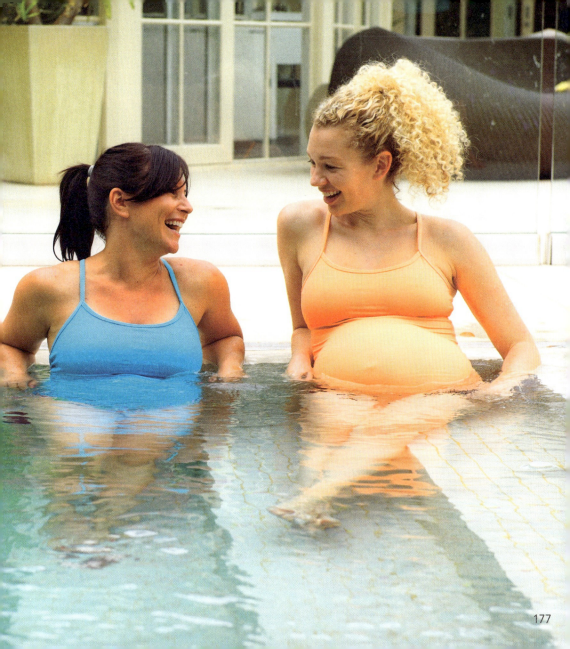

Chest-deep cardio and core

Movements such as jogging or walking in chest-deep water in a pool are much less stressful on your body than on land. You may find you are comfortable doing aqua aerobics-style exercise but always listen to your body. Maintain a moderate intensity and look after your pelvic joints by avoiding wide-based leg movements and exercises that load up one leg at a time. It is important to continue to sip water throughout water exercise, just as you would during land-based exercise.

Chest, back and core conditioning

- Stand in chest-deep water.
- Squat down so that your shoulders are under the water.
- Take your arms out wide to the side at shoulder height, palms facing forward.
- Engage your core and pelvic floor.
- Pull your hands through the water to bring your palms together.
- Now turn your palms outwards, thumbs down and push the water away, taking your arms wide again.

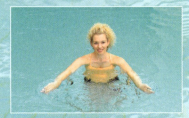

Arms by your side

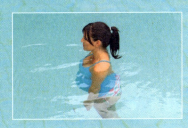

- Stand in chest-deep water.
- Squat down so that your shoulders are under the water, your arms by your side, one palm facing forwards, the other facing backwards.
- Engage your core and pelvic floor.
- Pull one arm forward and the other back (turning your palms to face in the direction of the movement).
- Feel like you are pulling and pushing the water.

Work your waist

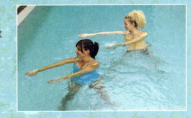

- Stand in chest-deep water with your feet hip-width apart.
- Squat down so that your shoulders are under the water.
- Raise your arms to chest height with the palms of your hands facing to the right.
- Engage your core and pelvic floor.
- Push both arms to the right rotating your upper body but keeping your pelvis and legs stable.
- Turn your palms and push your arms across your body to the left.
- Continue to push the water slowly from side to side focusing on working your waist while controlling your core.

Enjoy the support and resistance of an aqua workout.

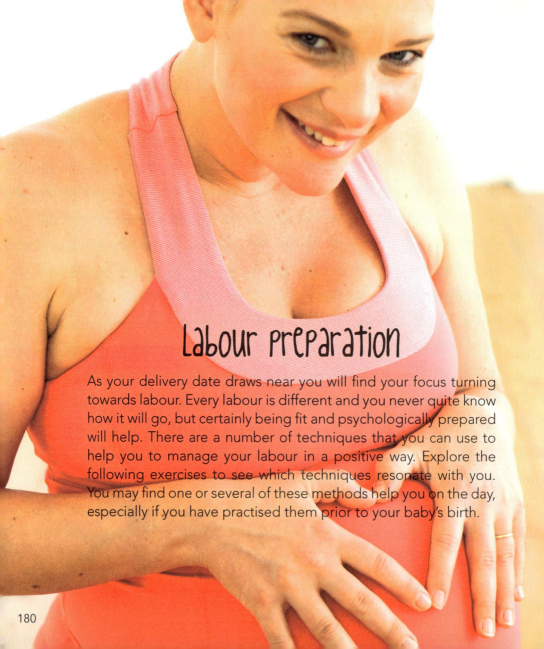

Labour preparation

As your delivery date draws near you will find your focus turning towards labour. Every labour is different and you never quite know how it will go, but certainly being fit and psychologically prepared will help. There are a number of techniques that you can use to help you to manage your labour in a positive way. Explore the following exercises to see which techniques resonate with you. You may find one or several of these methods help you on the day, especially if you have practised them prior to your baby's birth.

Contraction practice

Squats are used as a means of creating a physical discomfort for you to practise working with. Meanwhile, you will develop strong thighs, which is also handy during labour. Obviously the feeling of your quadriceps working when you squat is very different to labour pains, but it is a worthwhile exercise all the same.

There are two phases to your labour practice. The first is walking, simulating the time when you are between contractions. Walking also prevents stationary hypotension (light-headedness due to slow circulation), and reinforces the benefits of being upright and gently active during labour, whenever possible. Walk for a minute or two between your practice contractions. It is a time for focus, relaxation and reminding yourself of how well you are doing.

The second element is squatting while you practise various techniques to help you manage discomfort. Your squat can be with your feet hip-width apart, or wider if you have no hint of pelvic joint pain or incontinence. Remember to keep your weight in your heels and your back straight. Aim to squat for 30 seconds or more. As you get stronger build up to 60 seconds.

Practise the following labour preparation exercises in your third trimester. You can do these on their own or as a component of your workout. Five to 10 minutes practising one or a few of these techniques is plenty at any one time.

Working with your contractions and the time in between

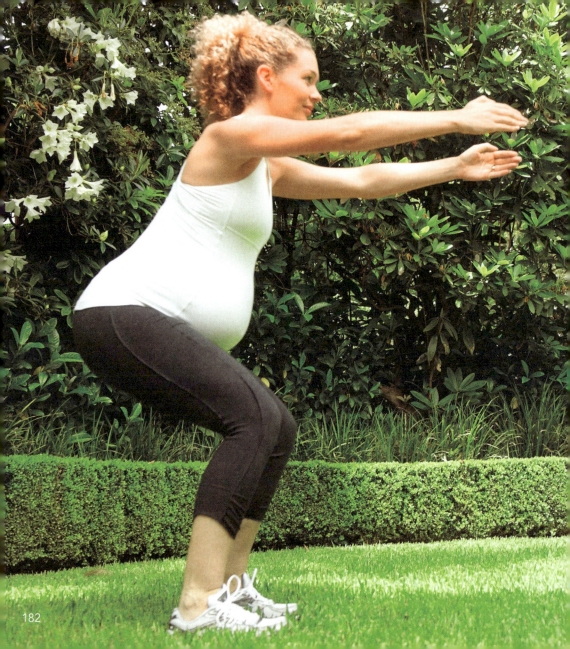

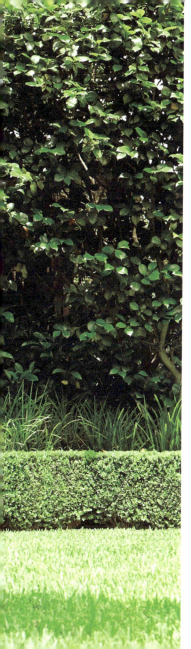

Welcome your contraction

Between contractions

- Walk around your room or garden and enjoy the freedom of walking and the ease in your body for a minute.
- Breathe calmly.

Contraction practice

- Stop walking and perform 5 slow squats.
- Now hold your squat at the bottom, with your weight in your heels.
- Perform small squats in this low 'seated' position.
- As you feel discomfort build up in your thighs welcome the contraction with a slow, deep breath.
- As you exhale, consciously relax your body and your breathing, telling yourself that 'this is good, every contraction brings me closer to meeting my new baby'.
- Focus on slow breaths as you squat for another 30 seconds.
- Stand up, shake out your legs as you say goodbye to the contraction with a slow, deep breath.

Between contractions

- Stand up and begin walking again, reminding yourself you will never see that contraction again.
- You are one contraction closer to meeting your new baby.

Work with your body and your baby

Contraction practice

- Stop walking and perform 5 slow squats.
- Hold your squat low.
- As the pain builds, greet your contraction with a slow, deep breath.
- Consciously relax your fingers, toes, neck and shoulders.
- Remind yourself that you do not want to tense your muscles when you feel pain, because you do not want to resist your labour.
- You will relax and allow your uterus to do its work.
- Breathe slowly and consciously relax your body to work with your uterus and your baby.

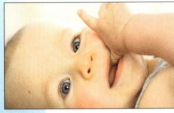

Between contractions

- Exhale as you stand up and say goodbye to that contraction.
- Begin walking again, reminding yourself how well you are working with your body and your baby.

Focus on your breath

Contraction practice

- As you move into your deep squat and you feel the discomfort in your thighs focus on your breath.
- Watch your breath flow in and out of your body.
- Watch it flow to your feet and away, down your back and back up, to your fingers and back up your arms.
- Relax with every exhale.

Between contractions

- Stand up and begin walking again, reminding yourself that you have prepared for this day, that you welcome this day and it is a short time in the big picture.

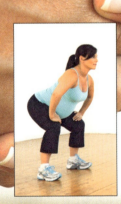

Place the pain to the back of your mind

Contraction practice

- Stop walking and perform 5 slow squats.
- Now hold your squat at the bottom, with your weight in your heels.
- As the pain builds up focus on your breath.
- Consciously acknowledge the pain but move it to the back of your mind – 'Yes it hurts, but it will not harm me'.
- Allow the pain to be there, at the back of your mind, doing it's work.
- Turning your conscious thought to another focus such as your breath, music, a visualisation, or counting.

Between contractions

- Say goodbye to that contraction with a big breath.
- You are one contraction closer to seeing your baby.
- Yes, it is getting harder but this is as expected.
- Feel proud of the wonderful job you are doing.

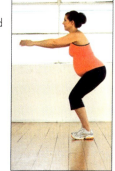

Your baby is working too

Contraction practice

- Stop walking and go into a low squat.
- Greet the contraction and relax your body with a deep sigh.
- Place the pain to the back of your mind and focus on your baby.
- Visualise their tiny little fingers and finger nails, their toes.
- Is your baby a boy or a girl? Do they have hair?
- Your baby is working too.
- Focus on your baby and remember why you are here and why you are working with your baby and your body.

Between contractions

- Shake your hands gently as you walk again.
- Take the time now to relax, to focus.
- Forget the last contraction, it is over.
- Do not think or worry about the next contraction.
- Now is the time to relax and re-energise.

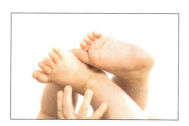

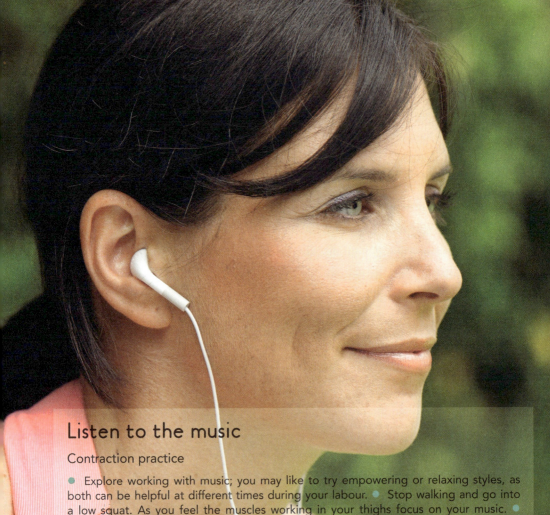

Listen to the music

Contraction practice

● Explore working with music; you may like to try empowering or relaxing styles, as both can be helpful at different times during your labour. ● Stop walking and go into a low squat. As you feel the muscles working in your thighs focus on your music. ● What instruments can you hear? ● Is this music you would like to take with you to your delivery? ● Listen to the rhythm. ● Walk and roll your shoulders up, back and down. This time between contractions is also a time to check your progress. ● Ask questions of your midwife or doctor so you are clear as to what stage you are up to in your labour.

Positive affirmations

Choose 1, 2 or 3 positive affirmations about you and your labour. Short simple positive statements in the present work best, for example:

- I am strong.
- I am working with my body and my baby.
- I trust my body.
- I am prepared for labour and motherhood.
- My body is in harmony with my uterus and my baby.
- I am relaxed, focused and empowered.

Contraction practice

- Choose one positive affirmation.
- As your contraction becomes stronger, move the pain to the back of your mind.
- Focus on your breath.
- Inside your head, in time with your breath, say your affirmation loudly and definitely several times over.

Between contractions

- Say goodbye to that contraction with a big breath.
- You are one contraction closer to seeing your baby.
- You are doing so well.

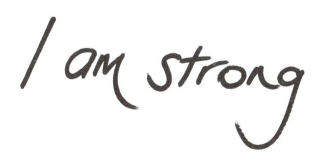

Stretch and mobilise

Mobility and flexibility exercises

Flexibility and mobility are important components of all fitness regimes; they are equally valuable during pregnancy. Including good stretching and mobilising exercises into your workout will promote your flexibility, healthy free-flowing movement and help you maintain an injury-free body. Look after your joints by stretching sensibly and within your comfort zone, taking care to avoid over-stretching or extreme movements. Hold your stretch at the point where you feel slight muscle tightness and breathe naturally.

Mobility goes hand in hand with flexibility and is a welcome addition to a pregnancy cool down. You will find the rhythmical rocking movements assist release of tension, freedom of movement and so are the perfect complement to the following stretches.

Top to toe

- Stand, holding your ball at the wall, at chest height.
- Walk forward as you roll the ball up the wall until you are stretching your arms up high.
- Walk in under the ball to feel a lovely stretch through your arms, shoulders and body.
- Hold for 5 slow breaths, roll the ball back down and repeat 3 times.

Upper back stretch

- Sitting or walking on the spot.
- Clasp your hands together and stretch them forward at chest height, palms facing away.
- Avoid shrugging your shoulders.
- Feel the stretch across your upper back.
- Hold for 5 slow breaths.
- Now reach your arms above your head, release your hands and allow them to float back down by your side.
- Repeat 3 times.

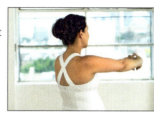

Calf Stretch

- Standing tall, take a step backwards with your right foot.
- Place your right heel to the floor.
- Bend your left knee as you lean forward.
- Feel the stretch in your right calf muscles.
- Hold for 10 slow breaths then slowly bring your feet together.
- Perform 3 pelvic tilts then step your left foot back to stretch your left calf.

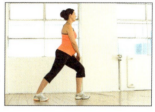

Upright chest stretch

- Sitting or walking on the spot.
- Bring your arms forward and together at chest height, palms facing upwards.
- Draw your shoulder blades downwards.
- Now open your arms taking your hands back at shoulder height.
- Feel a gentle stretch across your chest and shoulders.
- Hold for 10 slow breaths then relax your arms by your side.
- Repeat twice.

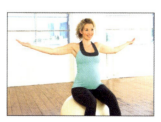

Neck stretch

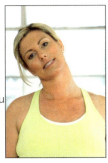

- Sit or stand tall.
- Draw your shoulder blades downwards and lengthen your neck.
- Looking straight ahead, tilt your head to the right taking your ear towards your right shoulder.
- At the same time push your left shoulder gently down as though you are holding a heavy suitcase in your left hand.
- Hold the stretch for 5 slow breaths then relax, roll your shoulders back and down 3 times then stretch the second side.
- Repeat twice.

Triceps stretch

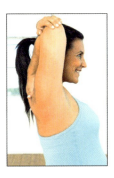

- Sitting or walking on the spot.
- Reach one arm high beside your ear.
- Bend the elbow so your hand is behind your head.
- Now use your other hand to gently push down on your elbow until you feel a slight stretch down the back of your arm.
- Keep your neck straight.
- Hold for 10 slow breaths and then repeat on the other arm.

Heaven and earth

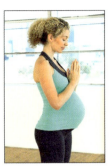

- Seated or standing, place your palms together in front of your chest.
- Inhale as you lift your right hand to your ear, to the sky, and press your left hand towards the floor.
- Look down your left arm and lean slightly to the left.
- Feel the stretch through your right arm and side.
- Hold for 5 breaths then return to prayer position ready to stretch to the other side.
- Repeat twice.

Seated rotation

- Sit tall on a fitball or slightly forward on a chair.
- Turn to the right, reaching your left hand across to the outside of your left knee.
- Turn as far as you can within comfort and hold for 5 slow breaths.
- Turn to the other side.
- Repeat twice.

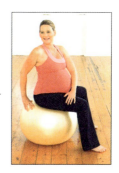

Upright back roll

- Stand in a narrow squat position, or sitting on a ball.
- Hands rest on your thighs to support your back.
- Lean forward with a straight back then round your back and slowly roll back to upright posture.
- Repeat 5 times.

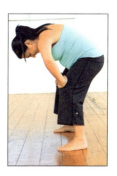

Fitball hamstring stretch

- Sit slightly forward on the ball, with your feet a little wider than your hips.
- Hands resting on your thighs.
- Lean forward and roll the ball backwards until you feel a slight stretch in the back of your legs.
- Hold for 10 slow breaths and then slowly roll back to upright sitting.
- Repeat twice.

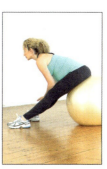

Standing hamstring stretch
- Place your right heel forward.
- Rest both hands on your left thigh to support your body.
- Now bend your left hip and knee as you incline your body forward until you feel a stretch in the back of your right leg.
- Hold for 10 slow breaths and then roll slowly back to standing.
- Stand up and perform 4 pelvic tilts before stretching the other side.
- Replace with fitball hamstring stretch if you have pelvic joint pain.

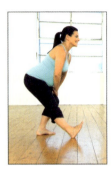

Standing lean and rock
- Stand facing the wall, with your feet slightly wider than your hips and your knees slightly bent.
- Lean forward with your forearms resting on the wall at chest height and your forehead resting on your hands.
- Slowly rock your pelvis from side to side.

Seated hip stretch
Some love this exercise others do not. If in doubt leave it out. Stretching the back of your hip in this way helps alleviate pelvic joint discomfort for some women
- Sit on a fitball with your hands by your hips, resting on the ball.
- Raise one foot off the floor.
- Carefully cross it over your thigh and then lower your knee downwards.
- Now roll the ball slightly back and lean forward until your feel a stretch in the back of your hip and buttocks.
- Hold this for 10 breaths then sit up, roll your back in a circle before repeating on the other leg.
- If this stretch feels too unsteady or you do not have a fitball you can perform a similar stretch sitting forward on a stable chair or couch, leaning forward over your crossed leg, or replace it with seated back and butt stretch.

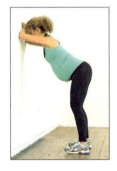

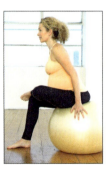

Seated back and butt stretch

- Sit forward on your fitball, feet a little wider than your hips.
- Keep your back straight and lean forward.
- Rest your elbows on your thighs.
- Slowly roll the ball back to increase the stretch.
- Hold for 10 slow breaths then roll back up to sitting.
- If you do not have a ball you can lean forward sitting on a stable chair.

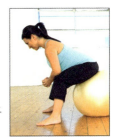

Kneeling back stretch

- Kneeling on the floor, place your hands on the floor in front.
- Sit back over your heels.
- Hold this arm- and back-stretch for 5 slow breaths then roll slowly back to upright kneeling.
- Repeat 3 times.

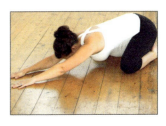

Kneeling lats stretch

- Kneeling on the floor reach your right arm forward and across your body to place it on the floor in front of your left shoulder.
- Now slowly sit back over your right heel.
- You should feel a lovely stretch through your right arm and side of your body.
- Hold for 10 slow breaths, then change sides.

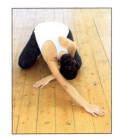

Kneeling pec stretch

- Kneel with the fitball arm's length from your side.
- Rest your hand on the ball.
- Place your other hand on the floor.
- Lower your chest towards the floor and turn away from the ball as though you are 'listening' to the floor.
- You should feel a gentle stretch across your chest and front of shoulder.
- Hold for 10 slow breaths, roll back to upright kneeling then change sides.

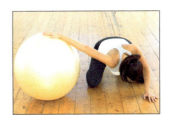

Rock and Roll

- Kneel on the floor with your forearms resting across the ball and your head resting on your hands.
- Make sure your knees are far enough away from the ball that your back is flat.
- Slowly rock the ball from side to side, rotating your thoracic spine.
- Ease away the tension in your back as you roll one elbow then the other towards the floor.
- Rock slowly side to side 10 times.

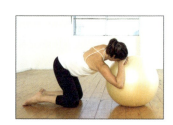

Kneeling circle

- Kneel on the floor with your chest and arms resting on the ball and your chin resting on your hands.
- Make sure your knees are far enough away from the ball that your back is flat.
- Slowly roll the ball to the side, forward, other side and back to roll your body in a horizontal circle. Imagine drawing a circle with your navel.
- Feel the release and relaxation in your back.
- Rotate 10 circles each way.

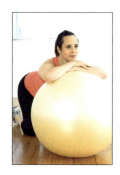

Quads stretch

- Lie on your side with your bottom knee slightly bent for balance.
- Bend your top knee to bring your foot behind you.
- Hold your ankle and push your hip slightly forward to feel a stretch down the front of your thigh.
- Hold for 10 slow breaths.
- Keep your knees bent and together and your feet on the floor as you roll over to stretch the other leg.

Relaxation

Relaxation is invaluable during pregnancy, not only to rest and release tension on a daily basis. Relaxation can be a powerful tool during labour and an excellent tonic for your body and mind during the busy times of early motherhood. Practise any of the following relaxation exercises when you are resting. Peaceful music will enhance your ability to calm your body and quieten your mind. If you practice relaxation to the same music, you may find the music eventually creates an almost immediate relaxation response both for you and your baby.

As you begin

- Make yourself comfortable lying on your side or sitting comfortably with your neck and shoulders supported.
- Sink into your position as you focus on your soft peaceful music.
- Take three slow deep breaths consciously allowing any tension to leave your body.

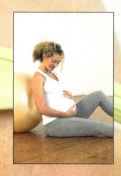

Slow your breath

- Let every part of your body sink into its resting position.
- Focus on slow deep breaths, breathing in through your nose and out gently through your lips as though blowing lightly through a straw.
- In time with your breath, count in 1,2,3,4 and out 1,2,3,4.
- With every exhalation relax your body a little more.
- Now counting at the same speed lengthen your breath, to breathe in for 5 and out for 5.
- Repeat this new longer breath 3 times, feeling the release and relaxation with every breath.
- Now make it slower and deeper, in for 6 and out for 6.
- And when you are comfortable in for 6 and out for 7 making your exhalation slower and longer.
- Continue slow deep breaths, allowing them to wash over your body as you relax deeper and deeper.
- When you are ready, slowly move your hands and feet, then your arms and legs. Take several minutes to gradually awaken and move back to an upright position.
- Sitting or standing, take three cleansing breaths, reaching for the sky and circling your arms back down with each one.

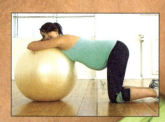

Give your breath a calming colour

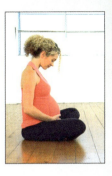

- Slow your breath to become slow and deep.
- Give your breath a colour that you find calm and peaceful.
- Now watch your breath flow in through your body to your toes.
- As you exhale see your breath flow out and away leaving your feet and legs relaxed.
- Watch your breath flow down your spine to your tailbone.
- Continue taking the soft, relaxing color to each part of your body.
- Give yourself permission to do absolutely nothing.
- When you are ready to come back, give your breath a colour that you find refreshing.
- Take cleansing breaths through your body, slowly moving your body in the way it is asking you to until you are ready to gradually kneel, sit and stand.
- Roll your shoulders and take a big breath in as you stretch to the sky

Visualisation — butterfly in the ferns

Visualisations can be very powerful relaxation techniques
- Settle into your position and close your eyes.
- Let the gentle music ease through your body.
- Slow your breath and consciously allow any tension to leave your body.
- Relax every muscle, your legs, arms, back, chest.
- Relax your jaw, your forehead and your face.
- Now take yourself in your mind to a small clearing in a beautiful rainforest.
- The space is clean, warm and fresh.
- This is a place you visit often, a place you know well.
- The only thing you ever do here is relax.
- Make yourself comfortable there, on the soft velvet like grass.
- Consciously slow your breath and settle into your special space in the lush green rainforest.
- Look around you and breathe in the beauty of nature.
- Surrounding your space are green ferns. On their delicate green leaves are small droplets of water.
- Amongst the ferns are the deep brown, strong trunks of the rainforest trees. They reach way above to the sky.
- At the top is the green canopy of the rainforest.
- Rays of sunlight are filtering through the trees, bringing their warmth and soft light to your special place.
- The sunlight is glistening on the droplets of water on the leaves of the ferns.
- Amongst the ferns are tiny, bright blue butterflies.
- They are flittering among the ferns, happy to be there with you.
- They are light, bright and beautiful and they haven't a worry in the world.
- As you gaze, you become the butterfly.
- You are light, bright and beautiful.
- Stay here, relaxing in your beautiful rainforest clearing
- Taking in the clean, warm air
- When you are ready, come back to where you are resting now.
- Start to move slowly, very gradually to your hands and knees, then kneeling and slowly back to sitting.
- The most beautiful thing about your rainforest clearing is you can go there whenever you like.

Getting ready for B-day

Labour is called labour not picnic for a reason! You can prepare physically and psychologically for the work that lies ahead in several ways.

Being familiar with the stages of labour gives you the ability to understand where you're at and so be able to pace yourself and make decisions about what you want or need.

During the first stage of labour, your uterus is contracting to gradually dilate your cervix. This is usually the longest stage, during which you will be working with your contractions. Labour management techniques will help you manage this stage, especially if you have practised them in the weeks prior. It is beneficial to resist natural responses to pain such as muscle tension or holding your breath. Underlying fitness, staying focused, relaxation techniques, mind-over-matter methods, visualisations, plus various movements and positions will help you assist, rather than resist, your labour's progress.

Towards the end of this first stage is a time known as transition. It is an intense phase, and while this might be challenging it is good to recognise and remind yourself that you are doing really well. Knowing that you are nearly there will give you the confidence to continue practising relaxation and working with your baby rather than fighting the contractions.

After transition, when your cervix is fully (10 centimetres) dilated it will be time to push. You will then work with your uterus to assist moving your baby through the birth canal.

After your baby is born you will continue to have contractions and the third stage of labour is the delivery of your placenta.

Physical and mental preparation

Exercising sensibly during your pregnancy will not necessarily make your labour shorter or less intense but it will certainly boost your fitness and endurance, allowing you to manage the physical demands and work with your body. Practising specific exercises such as squats and delivery positions will assist your strength for an active labour (see pages 181–185 for labour exercises). Rehearsing affirmative attitudes and techniques will empower you to feel positive, strong and ready for the big day.

Working with your body and baby
The usual response to pain is to brace yourself, tense up and hold your breath. All of these things might hinder the progress of your labour so practising the techniques below can help.

Different positions
Explore different positions for labour, as you never know which one will appeal on the day. Rhythmical movements such as rocking and swaying are also popular.

Relaxation techniques
Relaxation techniques on page 195 can be used at any time during your pregnancy, or thereafter, but may be particularly useful, especially if you have practised them, during labour. Focusing on your breath, colour, and visualisations are all popular as well as massage and aromatherapy. Many women enjoy the warmth and relief of warm water in a shower or bath.

Music soothes

Music can be helpful during labour, gentle calming music will complement your relaxation techniques. If you use the same peaceful music when you are practising your relaxation daily, prior to labour, it can be very powerful on the day. You may like to select empowering, uplifting music for other times during your labour.

Positive affirmations

Positive affirmations can also be incredibly powerful, even more so if you have been working with these beforehand as on page 187.

Other forms of pain management

Other forms of pain management include TENS machines, and medical options. It is important to get a sound understanding of these from an unbiased professional. Whilst you may feel you want to avoid nitrous oxide (laughing gas), medication or an epidural, you may change your mind on the day and having sound prior knowledge will help you make an informed decision on the day.

Your labour kit bag

Every woman is different and every approach to birthing your baby will be different. Make sure you explore all the options available to you for helping you through labour. A number of the options listed in the kit bag will need a bit of practice beforehand. For example, you might want to include visualisation techniques or positive affirmations in your exercise program. Following are some suggestions for including in your own labour kit bag.

- Different positions for birthing
- Rhythmical movements to help you ride through your contractions
- Relaxation
- Visualisation
- Music (empowering and relaxing) will help you to relax
- Positive affirmations
- Massage
- Aromatherapy – a selection of oils to put you in a calm frame of mind
- Hot packs for aching backs
- Medical assistance such at TENS machines for pain management. Discuss options with your healthcare provider to help you make informed decisions on the day.

Early days of motherhood

After the exciting arrival of your gorgeous bundle of joy you are likely to feel elated, excited, delighted and overwhelmed by emotions. Every new mother's experience is different. Your comfort levels, energy levels and need for rest will vary significantly according to your pre-existing fitness and your labour. While many women are keen to get their body back in shape, now is not the time to rush into doing too much, too soon. Magazine articles that illustrate how famous women are back in their pre-baby jeans soon after delivery create inappropriate and unrealistic expectations. It took you 9 months for your body to change and gain weight. Trying to diet or exercise too early can lead to more strain, incontinence and emotional stress. Instead it is a time to settle into motherhood, rejoice in the arrival of your new baby and allow your body to recover after pregnancy and delivery.

- During the first few days after delivery rest up, being sure to have plenty of time off your feet and allowing your body to recover.
- During the first week you can recommence pelvic floor and gentle indrawing abdominal core exercises.
- Walking, pelvic floor, core and postural focus is plenty for the early weeks while you are settling into breastfeeding and life with a new baby.

For further advice on how to progress your fitness sensibly from day one to a year after delivery, and exercise to help you recover and regain your fitness as a new mum, check out my companion book, *New Mums Shape Up*.

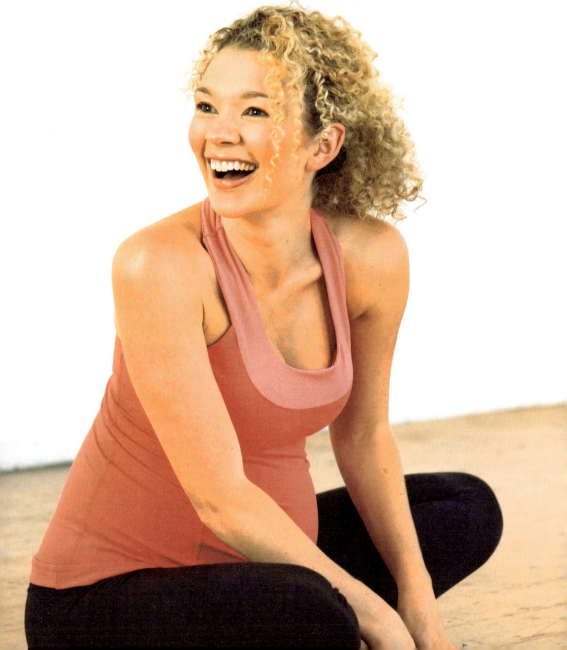

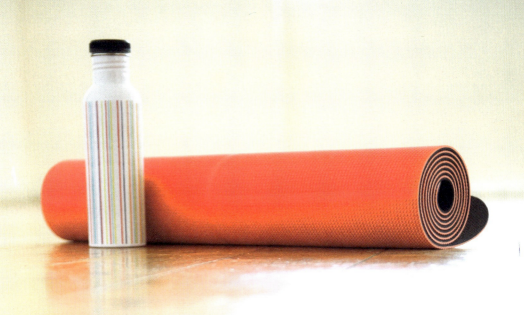

PART FOUR
THE EXERCISE PROGRAMS

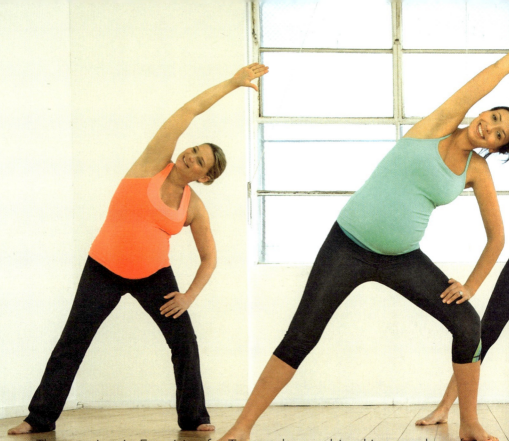

The exercises in *Exercising for Two* can be combined in a number of ways. Create your own custom-designed prenatal workout to suit your goals and abilities, or select from one of the following physiotherapy designed pregnancy exercise regimes. The programs vary in their levels and style, providing options for women at all stages of their pregnancy and fitness levels.

You will find programs for women needing to take it easy, and those who can work a little harder. Suggestions for each trimester and the different training focus are all included.

Remember to vary your training and honour the importance of rest and relaxation at this important and precious time of your life.

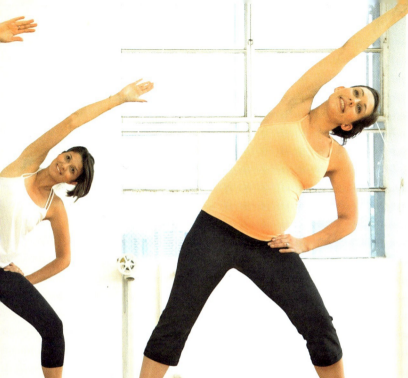

Exercising for two programs

The following programs will help you in selecting and designing your own prenatal exercise programs to suit your goals and individual situation.

Program basics:

- It is important to vary your pelvic floor training styles. Choose from the pelvic floor exercises on pages 92–97.
- Labour practice and relaxation: Mix and match options each workout.
- The perfect finale for any exercise session is to include stretching and gentle mobilising exercises. Choose from the options on pages 188–194 to suit.
- How often you exercise depends on what else is going on in your life. If you have time and energy 3 to 5, 15 to 45 minute, exercise sessions per week is good. How long and how energetic depends on your fitness and wellbeing. It is important to listen to your body and balance your daily life, exercise and rest. Varying your programs, within the framework of your ability, will help to keep your interest high and stress on your body low.
- Check you are following sensible exercise guidelines as recommended in this book and by your healthcare provider.

1 When rest is best – for gentle joint and muscle maintainance

Gentle moves will help your muscle tone, joint mobility and circulation. A good choice for women who need to rest up or a perfect lighter option for those who want to take it easy.

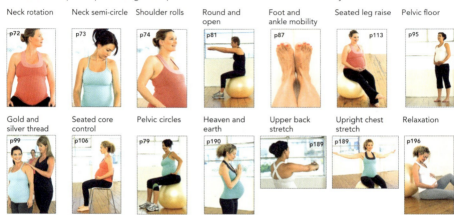

Neck rotation p72 · Neck semi-circle p73 · Shoulder rolls p74 · Round and open p81 · Foot and ankle mobility p87 · Seated leg raise p113 · Pelvic floor p95

Gold and silver thread p99 · Seated core control p106 · Pelvic circles p79 · Heaven and earth p190 · Upper back stretch p189 · Upright chest stretch p189 · Relaxation p196

2 Starting out – gentle exercises for the first trimester

A safe and sensible choice for those who have been recently inactive or who need to take it easy.

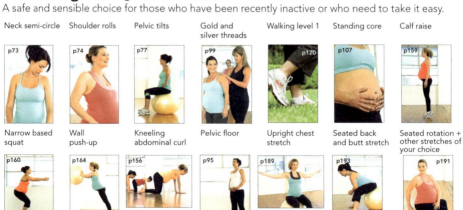

Neck semi-circle p73 · Shoulder rolls p74 · Pelvic tilts p77 · Gold and silver threads p99 · Walking level 1 p120 · Standing core p107 · Calf raise p159

Narrow based squat p160 · Wall push-up p164 · Kneeling abdominal curl p156 · Pelvic floor p95 · Upright chest stretch p189 · Seated back and butt stretch p193 · Seated rotation + other stretches of your choice p191

3 1st trimester workout – for active women during the first sixteen weeks

Appropriate options for if you have been exercising prior to pregnancy, are feeling fit and well and have the all clear to continue exercising.

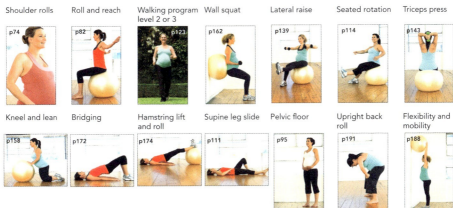

4 2nd trimester, taking it easy – a slow and steady start

For mum and bub in the second trimester who have been unable to exercise until now.

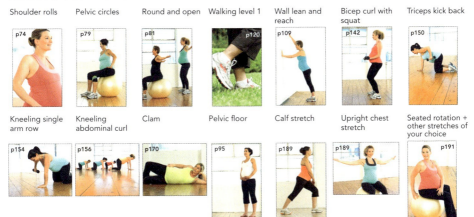

5 2nd trimester workout – keeping strong and taking care

For women who are fit and well and continuing a sensible prenatal fitness program.

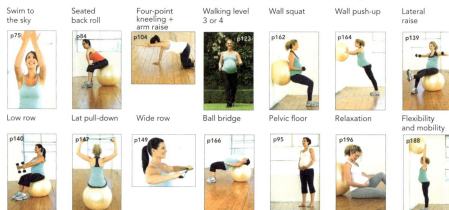

6 3rd trimester workout – staying strong as you grow

A program of safe and effective options as your delivery date comes closer.

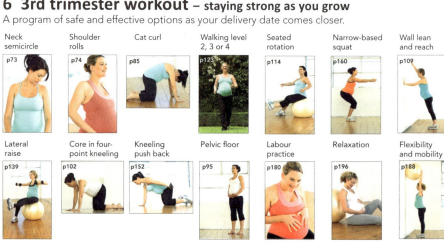

7 Protect your pelvic joints – helping to manage or prevent pain
A specific program for women experiencing or concerned about pelvic joint pain.

Shoulder rolls	Pelvic tilts	Seated back roll	Fitball heel digs	Seated rotation	Seated semi squat	Seated leg raise
p74	p77	p84	p132	p114	p145	p113

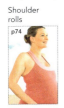 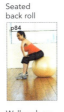 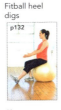 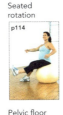 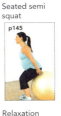 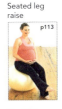

Lat pull down	Triceps press	Wall push up	Clam	Pelvic floor	Relaxation	Flexibility and mobility
p147	p143	p164	p170	p95	p196	p188

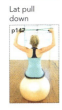 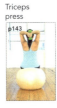 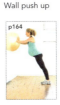

8 Fitball fitness – get on the ball
Fabulous training tool throughout your pregnancy.

Pelvic circles	Roll and reach	Seated leg raise	Fitball wall hover	Fitball march	Fitball heel digs	Seated step touch
p79	p82	p113	p115	p131	p132	p133

     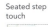

Lateral raise	Wall push up	Wall squat	Top to toe	Ball bridge	Pelvic floor	Kneeling circle + other flexibility and mobility options
p139	p164	p162	p188	p166	p95	p194

9 Water workout – for minimal stress, optimal results
Enjoy this safe and effective aqua-based program.

| Swim to the sky p75 | Neck rotation p72 | Seated rotation p114 | Swimming level 1, 2 or 3 p128 | Deep water running p176 | Chest back and core conditioning p178 | At the wall p176 |

| Arms by your side p179 | Work your waist p179 | At the wall p176 | Standing core p107 | Pelvic floor long holds p93 | Upper back stretch p189 | Upright chest stretch p189 |

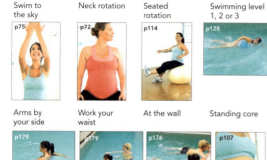
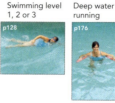
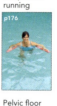

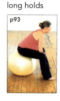

10 Focus on your core and pelvic floor – build inner strength
The pelvic floor and core exercises in this program are vital foundations for all active mums-to-be.

| Round and open p81 | Gold and silver threads p99 | Pelvic floor strong holds p94 | Seated leg raise p113 | Pelvic circles p79 | Pelvic floor long holds p93 | Seated rotation p114 |

| Fitball wall hover p115 | Core in four-point kneeling p102 | Pelvic floor long hold + quick lifts p96 | Kneel and lean p158 | Relax your pelvic floor p97 | Rock and roll p194 | Kneeling circle p194 |

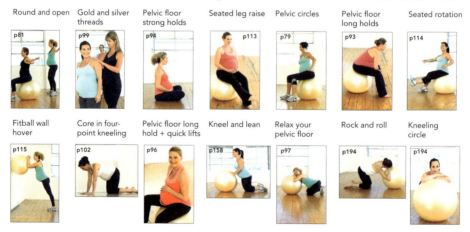

11 Upper body strength – develop strong arms and fabulous posture
A program to focus on your arms, chest and back for strength and upright stance.

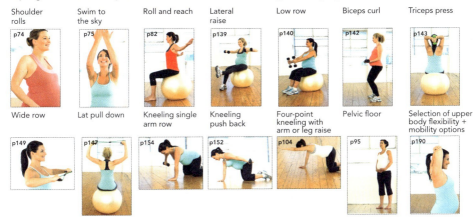

Shoulder rolls — p74
Swim to the sky — p75
Roll and reach — p82
Lateral raise — p139
Low row — p140
Biceps curl — p142
Triceps press — p143

Wide row — p149
Lat pull down — p147
Kneeling single arm row — p154
Kneeling push back — p152
Four-point kneeling with arm or leg raise — p104
Pelvic floor — p95
Selection of upper body flexibility + mobility options — p190

12 Lower body strength – strong thighs, strength and definition
Strong muscles below the belt not only look great but will also help you during labour and help you with all the extra carrying and lifting you will be doing as a new mum.

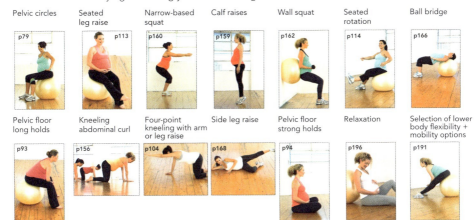

Pelvic circles — p79
Seated leg raise — p113
Narrow-based squat — p160
Calf raises — p159
Wall squat — p162
Seated rotation — p114
Ball bridge — p166

Pelvic floor long holds — p93
Kneeling abdominal curl — p156
Four-point kneeling with arm or leg raise — p104
Side leg raise — p168
Pelvic floor strong holds — p94
Relaxation — p196
Selection of lower body flexibility + mobility options — p191

13 Preparing for labour – strengthen your body and prepare your mind
These exercises will help you to practice and prepare for labour and early motherhood.

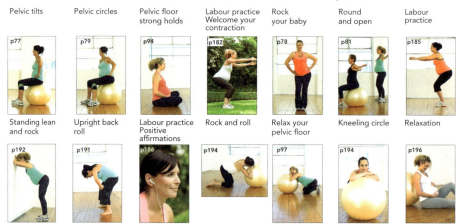

14 Early days of motherhood – time to rest, recover and rejoice
To allow your body several days of rest and then gradually commence gentle moves over the following weeks to help your body slowly recover. Do not rush back to too much too soon.

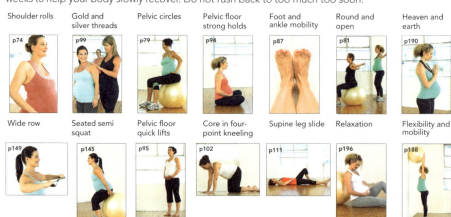

Thank You

I must be the most fortunate person in the world. I have so many wonderful people to thank for their advice, support and inspiration in the creation of *Exercising for Two*. Firstly, my women's health mentor and guru, Dr Margaret Sherburn, who inspired me to start teaching exercise classes for pregnant women twenty years ago and has so generously shared her knowledge, advice and encouragement ever since. Many other women's health physiotherapists have leant me their ear and wise thoughts, but two in particular deserve special mention: Thank you to Janetta Webb for her loyal friendship and invaluable advice and feedback, especially with regards to pelvic floor; and to Shira Kramer, once an enthusiastic student and now a sensational support, always ready to discuss a point, lend a hand and challenge my thoughts – thanks Shira, not only for your encouragement and ongoing assistance, but also for helping me find the most delightful and photogenic pregnant women. Thanks to all my encouraging fitness colleagues, especially Jenny Schembri-Portelli for her positive attitude and her invaluable input on aqua exercise. A special thank you to Nigel Champion and everyone at the Australian Fitness Network for their continued support. To the special women who brought their tummies and their beautiful smiles to be photographed and who made *Exercising for Two* come alive; thank you Marie, Lauren, Lee, Mel, Ashleigh, Leigh, Lisa, Stef and Bree. I wish you all the best for the next, very exciting, stage of your lives. Thanks, too, to lululemon athletica and Brooks for helping the girls look great. Bronwyn Kidd, you are a magician behind the lens. Thank you for your creative and beautiful photography. And to designer Jude Rowe, who put the words and pictures together with delightful flair and finesse. My gratitude too, to all at Hachette, especially Helen Littleton, who had faith in *Exercising for Two* from the beginning. Thank you for your creativity, editing skills, patience and support and for allowing me to be involved in every element of this book's creation. My gorgeous family Dave, Dan and Jess, for your tolerance and patience, and Megan and Belinda, who again helped me to keep the home fires burning. A huge thank you to Stef, for her role on both sides of the camera, her sensational productions skills, tireless advice, support, encouragement, and, above all, her friendship. Most importantly, thank you to all the wonderful pregnant women whom I've had the joy to meet. It is you, your thoughts and your experiences that inspired this book.

About the author

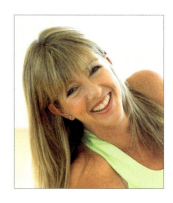

Lisa Westlake is a mother of two, a physiotherapist, a highly regarded fitness instructor and an international presenter. She lectures in several Melbourne universities and is involved in promoting community health and well-being through her writing, ABC Radio health and fitness segments and hosting community fun run and walk events such as the Mother's Day Classic and the Brazilian Butterfly Queen of the Lake. Through her business, Physical Best, Lisa combines her knowledge and skills in both physiotherapy and fitness to provide exercise programs for people of all ages and abilities. Alongside her passion for helping women achieve their physical and emotional best, Lisa has drawn on over 20 years' experience of instructing prenatal fitness classes to bring a wealth of knowledge and information to *Exercising for Two*. Lisa has produced 6 fitness DVDs, and has presented in numerous countries on all things health and fitness, and her first two books, *Strong to the Core* and *Strong and Stable* have been published in many countries. Lisa was awarded Australian Fitness Instructor of the Year in 2000, Australian Fitness Presenter of the Year in 2003 and Australian Fitness Author of the Year in 2009.